P9-BYF-319

WOULD YOU PUT HOT PEPPER ON SORE MUSCLES?

You can find out by looking up *CAYENNE*!

As easy as using an English dictionary, DICTIONARY OF NATURAL HEALING provides fast, reliable answers to your questions about natural remedies. So if you are wondering . . .

- CAN DIFFERENT COLORS INFLUENCE MY MOOD . . . OR EVEN MY BLOOD PRESSURE? Check out *COLOR THERAPY* and you may begin feeling "in the pink."

- WHAT'S THE FUSS ABOUT *ESSENTIAL FATTY ACIDS*? This entry tells you why you need them, where to get them, and how they help *lower* cholesterol.

- IS THE *HAY DIET* FOR PEOPLE . . . OR HORSES? Discover this fascinating approach to combining certain kinds of foods at the same meal to alleviate arthritis, digestive disorders and obesity.

READ ON TO FIND OUT THE OTHER SURPRISING
WAYS NATURAL REMEDIES CAN WORK
FOR YOU . . .

DICTIONARY OF
NATURAL HEALING

DICTIONARY of NATURAL HEALING

PL - 3790 - 2344

DEBORAH R. MITCHELL

A Lynn Sonberg Book

St. Martin's Paperbacks

NOTE: If you purchased this book without a cover you should be aware that this book is stolen property. It was reported as "unsold and destroyed" to the publisher, and neither the author nor the publisher has received any payment for this "stripped book."

DICTIONARY OF NATURAL HEALING

Copyright © 1998 by Lynn Sonberg.

All rights reserved. No part of this book may be used or reproduced in any manner whatsoever without written permission except in the case of brief quotations embodied in critical articles or reviews. For information address St. Martin's Press, 175 Fifth Avenue, New York, NY 10010.

ISBN: 0-312-96516-8

Printed in the United States of America

St. Martin's Paperbacks edition / September 1998

St. Martin's Paperbacks are published by St. Martin's Press, 175 Fifth Avenue, New York, NY 10010.

10 9 8 7 6 5 4 3 2 1

A Note to Readers

This book is for informational purposes only. Readers are advised to consult a trained medical professional before acting on any of the information in this book. The fact that a particular therapy, treatment, herb or supplement is discussed in the book does not mean that the author or publisher recommend its use. Similarly, the fact that an organization is listed in Appendix A to the book does not mean that the author or publisher recommend any of the therapies, treatments, herbs or supplements they may offer or suggest.

Contents

Appendixes

Introduction

Welcome to the exciting world of natural medicine. You, along with millions of other Americans of all ages, ethnic backgrounds, philosophical beliefs, and economic statuses are seeking out, learning about, and enjoying the benefits of natural healing techniques. This book can be your guide to this evolving world of medicine and help you find your way among the many advantages it has to offer.

If you picked up this book thinking it's going to read like a standard dictionary—ho hum, boring—you'll be pleasantly surprised to find that you're wrong. First of all, *Dictionary of Natural Healing* provides you with the most up-to-date, comprehensive information on natural medicine in an easy-to-read format not available in other books on the market. The term "natural healing" here refers to those techniques, remedies, or terms that *complement* the practice of conventional medicine. Holistic medicine treats a person as a whole, taking into account his or her physical, emotional, and spiritual states of being. Natural medicine's aim is to prevent health problems, promote well-being and vitality, and treat ailments. Thus all of the entries in this *Dictionary* have been selected with these purposes in mind.

Furthermore, within seconds of thinking of a therapy or herb, you can turn to the desired term and have at your fingertips a concise definition, alternative terms, the therapeutic uses of the therapy or remedy, and a brief description of how the therapy or remedy works. All the information comes from well-researched sources, including leaders in the field of natural medicine. No regular dictionary can offer you this scope of information.

What the *Dictionary* is *not* is a "how-to" book. The entries are not cluttered with prescriptive information, details on how to prepare or administer remedies, or how a particular therapy is conducted. However, *Dictionary* is a handy guide to help you find more information about any technique or remedy that has piqued your interest. After reading the entry for **polarity therapy**, for example, you may want to know more: Where can I find a practitioner? What goes on during a typical therapy session? What other literature can I get on this topic?

To find such details in other sources, refer to the appendixes. The first appendix, *Organizations and Resources*, is a list of names, addresses, and phone numbers of organizations and other information services that provide practitioner referrals and in-depth details about particular therapies, remedies, or practices. In the second appendix, *Books, Periodicals, and Mail Order Sources*, you will find a wealth of written and audiovisual resources that can answer your questions and satisfy your curiosity. In addition, we have included "ALSO SEE" sections at the ends of many entries, which lead you to other relevant entries.

This may well be the first dictionary you have ever enjoyed reading, and one you'll keep coming back to again and again for years to come. We wish you good health and happy browsing!

A

Acidophilus (as-uh-DAF-uh-les) is a form of bacteria, *Lactobacillus acidophilus*, that can help protect against some yeast infections (including candida), facilitate digestion of milk products, prevent indigestion, help fight gastrointestinal cancer, restore a healthy bacterial environment in the intestines, and help control cholesterol levels. It is also a general term for liquid or dried cultures of the bacteria.

Acidophilus occurs naturally in the body and is found in acidophilus milk and some yogurts (check the label for the words *Lactobacillus acidophilus* or *L. acidophilus*); powdered acidophilus supplements can be found in health food stores. Some nondairy varieties of acidophilus, which use carrot juice as a base, are also available. Women who experience frequent yeast infections and individuals who are taking antibiotics may benefit from adding acidophilus to their diet. In some cases, acidophilus helps control the diarrhea that is often associated with taking antibiotics.
ALSO SEE colon hydrotherapy

Aconite (AK-uh-nite) *(Aconitum napellus)* is a deadly plant that has excellent healing abilities when used as a homeopathic remedy. Also known as monkshood, friar's cap, and wolfsbane, aconite, which is a word derived from the Latin *acon*, or ''dart,'' was once used as a poison on the tips of hunters' arrows. Dr. Samuel Hahnemann, the father of **homeopathy**, added aconite to his remedy list in 1805 and used it to treat people who had fever or sudden severe pain.

Today, aconite is commonly used to treat infections and conditions that occur suddenly, such as colds and flu that affect people who are exposed to abrupt changes in the weather as well as people who experience intense emotional stress or panic attacks. Aconite is also effective in the treatment of: eye inflammation caused by injury, asthma, dry cough, sore throat, stiff neck, high temperature accompanied by great thirst, ringing of the ears, tonsillitis, teething, toothache, sleeplessness, animal bites, and types of abdominal pain that become worse when drinking cold water. Homeopaths often recommend taking aconite for severe, sudden, brief pain when people are unsure about what else to take.

For emotional problems, aconite is suggested as a homeopathic remedy for fear, anger, anxiety, grief, restlessness, and a sense of impending doom. It is often recommended for people who fear death because they are ill, or because they are in labor. Aconite may be helpful for people who are afraid to go to the dentist, who are about to undergo surgery, or who are agoraphobic.
ALSO SEE homeopathy

Acupoints (AK-yoo-points) are acupuncture points that lie along the **meridians** of the body. Each specific point, of which there are approximately 350, is associated with a particular body organ or system. Acupuncture needles are inserted in a particular point to enhance and improve the flow of **chi** (or *qi*) and restore balance and harmony to the body. Acupoint sites are also used during **moxibustion** and by acupressure therapists. Each acupoint has a specific name or designation, depending on the treatment modality to which it refers.
ALSO SEE acupuncture; acupressure; moxibustion

Acupressure (AK-yoo-presh-er) is the application of pressure, usually with the thumbs or fingers, to designated points on the body in an effort to release blocked energy and return internal balance to the body. Some people refer to acupressure as "acupuncture without the use of needles" because both acupressure and acupuncture are based on the same concept of health. That concept, according to ancient Chinese tradition, is that all people possess a life energy called **chi** (*chi* in Chinese; *qi* in Japanese) that flows through them along invisible pathways called **meridians**.

The free flow of chi is necessary for health and balance. When chi becomes blocked at various points in the body due to illness, trauma or injury, emotional stress, poor nutrition, or poor posture, the result can be disease, pain, or other symptoms. Those who practice acupressure believe that each one of the approximately 350 acupressure points that have been identified on the body is an energy conductor. Application of pressure to specific points called **acupoints**—sites chosen because they correspond to a particular complaint or ailment for which people seek help—can unblock "stalled" energy flow and provide relief.

People in China and Japan have enjoyed the benefits of acupressure for millennia, but this healing technique became popular in the United States only after President Nixon visited China in 1971. Since that time, many Americans have sought acupressure and **acupuncture** treatments from professionals or have learned how to do basic techniques on themselves and others. Acupressure is especially helpful in relieving pain, such as backache, arthritis, and headache, and other ailments, including asthma, constipation, fatigue, nausea, and motion sickness. A Japanese version of acupressure combined with massage, called **shiatsu**, has gained wide acceptance in the United States. Other variations of acupressure include: **shen tao**, which adds a spiritual aspect to acupressure; **do-in**, a form of self-shiatsu treatment that includes stretching movements; **amma massage**, which uses acupuncture points, as well as other points discovered by the therapy's founder, Tina Sohn; **tuina**, an ancient Chinese method of hands-on therapies; and **jin shin**

do, a body-mind approach that combines gentle yet deep finger pressure with verbal coaching to help release emotional and physical tension.

Acupuncture (AK-yoo-punk-cher) is the practice of inserting ultra-fine needles into specific spots on the body as a way to free-up blocked energy, restore balance to the body, and relieve pain. It has been practiced in China for about 2,000 years and in Japan for nearly 400 years.

Interest in acupuncture in the West has been more recent. Few Western doctors were interested in acupuncture during the late nineteenth century; it was not until President Nixon visited China in 1971 that acupuncture gained much significant attention in the West. At that time James Reston, a columnist for *The New York Times* who accompanied Nixon, underwent an emergency appendectomy and chose acupuncture instead of postoperative painkillers. Reston's praise of acupuncture opened up a wave of interest that is still growing.

According to traditional Chinese medicine, life energy called **chi** flows throughout the body along invisible "highways" called **meridians**. Scattered along these pathways, of which there are 14 major ones, are places where chi is near the skin surface. These sites are called **acupoints**. Once a practitioner has diagnosed where chi is blocked in the body, she or he can needle those points, which then influences the flow of chi and helps return balance to the body.

There are various forms of acupuncture, including classical or Five Element acupuncture, medical acupuncture, Japanese acupuncture, and **auricular therapy**. Some acupuncturists practice a variation in which they burn an herb called mugwort (a method called **moxibustion**) over selected acupuncture points or directly on the needles; others practice **electroacupuncture**, in which low-voltage electrical stimulation is applied to the needles. Both of these latter methods are believed to increase the effectiveness of treatment. Application of laser beams to acupuncture points is yet another new approach to acupuncture.

More than 20 years of medical research conducted around the world indicates that acupuncture works neuroelectrically. This means, explains George A. Ulett, M.D., Ph.D., director of the Department of Psychiatry at Deaconness Hospital in St. Louis, that the meridians are actually the motor nerves, which are connected to the body's major muscles. When needles are inserted into acupuncture points, they stimulate the bioelectrical energy that moves along the nerves and trigger the release of chemicals called neurotransmitters, particularly endorphins. These neurotransmitters are the body's natural painkillers.

Acupuncture has been successful in the treatment of headache, carpal tunnel syndrome, arthritis, sciatica, low back pain, fibromyalgia, asthma, depression, and narcotic addiction.

ALSO SEE acupressure; Chinese medicine

Acu-Yoga is a variation of yoga in which yoga positions are used to apply pressure to specific acupressure points against a floor or other nonyielding surface. It is a self-help therapy created by Michael Reed Gach, founder of the Acupressure Institute in Berkeley, California. Some of the positions work best when people lie with their fingertips pressed into the acupoints; others are effective if people lie on a tennis ball or similar round object in order to stimulate specific acupoints, especially on the back. Acu-Yoga is effective in the treatment of back and neck pain, headache, heartburn, impotency, menstrual cramps, and shoulder tension.

ALSO SEE acupressure

Alexander Technique is a comprehensive program of a series of simple movements that allow people to develop more control and awareness of daily activities. It is based on the concept that people unconsciously learn habits that interfere with their natural balance, coordination, and ability to function optimally. The Alexander Technique helps them replace dysfunctional movements and habits with healthier ones.

F. Matthais Alexander (1869-1955) was an actor who observed that many people perform everyday routine tasks, such as walking, lifting, brushing their teeth, and sitting, inefficiently. This occurs, he believed, because most people press their head back and down, which compresses the spine. This posture creates tension, hinders movement and flexibility, and results in pain, fatigue, poor posture, headache, and other complaints. Once this posture is corrected by "maintain[ing] the poise of the head on top of the lengthening spine in movement and at rest," people can enjoy more energy, release of tension, and greater flexibility.

The Alexander Technique is usually taught one-on-one by teachers (Alexander Technique practitioners refer to themselves as teachers rather than therapists) in sessions lasting from 30 to 60 minutes. Teachers introduce easy, nonstrenuous movements to help students gain conscious control of their physical behavior and to train the muscles to maintain good posture during daily routine activities. Because each individual has unique habits, Alexander Technique teachers tailor lessons to each person's needs.

In order for the Alexander Technique to be effective, participants need to increase their awareness of how they move during everyday activities and consciously correct it. The more aware they are of their physical habits and movements, the more likely their bodies will become reprogrammed to respond subconsciously with the new movements and postures. This takes time and daily practice.

Although the Alexander Technique does not treat specific ailments or symptoms, it can result in a significant improvement in overall health and well-being, increase flexibility and energy level, and allow people to eliminate habits that can cause them physical, emotional, and mental stress.
ALSO SEE Feldenkrais Method

Alfalfa is a common crop used to feed cattle and sheep and as a food supplement for humans. It was first cultivated around 1000 B.C. in the Middle East. Today the United States is the world's largest producer.

Alfalfa is regarded by some people as a powerful "green" food, reportedly effective for treatment of everything from constipation to intestinal ulcers, arthritis, hemorrhoids, bad breath, high blood pressure, and cancer. Although alfalfa does consist of 16 percent protein, various vitamins and minerals (particularly potassium, magnesium, calcium, iron, and vitamins A, E, D, and K), and eight enzymes associated with improved digestion, there is some concern over the use of alfalfa as a food or supplement. A report in the November 1995 issue of the *American Journal of Clinical Nutrition* noted that people who have diets high in alfalfa seed or sprouts or who take alfalfa tablets have a higher incidence of systemic lupus erythematosus and that taking alfalfa tablets may activate inactive lupus. Moderate, occasional consumption of alfalfa seeds or sprouts or a cup of alfalfa tea is considered safe, but alfalfa tablets may be toxic for some people.

Allium Cepa (Al-lee-um SEE-pa) is a homeopathic remedy prepared from the common red onion. It is most commonly used as an acute cold and cough remedy, especially when the following symptoms are present: excessive watering of the eyes; a bland, watery nasal discharge; sneezing; congestion or dull, frontal headache or, occasionally, a throbbing headache; and cough with tearing pain in the larynx that is worse in the evening. Symptoms are generally worse in warm environments and better in the open air except for cough, which may be worse from breathing in cold air. Because allium is used primarily as an acute remedy, no extensive psychological profile has been developed.
ALSO SEE homeopathy

Aloe Vera (AL-oh VER-uh) is a plant in the lily family with thick, cushiony leaves, which contain a gel-like substance that is valued for both its external and internal healing powers. There are about 300 species of aloe, but "true aloe" (aloe vera) is considered to be the most effective. It is a popular house plant in the United States and is most widely grown in the desert regions of Africa and the Mediterranean.

Aloe vera has been an important herb since about 1500 B.C., when the ancient Egyptians used it to treat skin problems. Alexander the Great reportedly fought for possession of an island off the coast of Africa so his soldiers would have access to an adequate supply of aloe vera to treat their wounds. Herbalists in many different cultures have used this herb to treat burns, rashes, wounds, and hemorrhoids.

A substance called allantoin, which accelerates wound healing, is believed to be partially responsible for aloe vera's effectiveness for external use. It also contains salicylates, the same pain-killing agents found in aspirin. Aloe vera is a natural moisturizer and may help to prevent wrinkles. Taken internally, it is a laxative and benefits liver function. Most recently it has been used to treat radiation burns.

Investigations into the use of aloe vera in the treatment of cancer, AIDS, and diabetes are ongoing. Several studies of its use in treating inflammatory bowel disease (including Crohn's disease and ulcerative colitis) find that aloe is a potent anti-inflammatory. In the veterinary arena, aloe vera injections can greatly improve the survival rate of cats with feline leukemia, and they appear to have antiviral effects against other feline viruses, such as feline AIDS, measles, and influenza.

ALSO SEE herbal medicine

Alphahydroxy Acids (al-fa-hi-DROX-ee), or AHAs, are acids derived from fruit juices, sour milk, fermented grapes, vegetables, and other plants, which are used to help reverse the aging process and treat skin disorders. Scientifically they are known as alpha keto/carboxylic acids.

Studies show that when concentrations of AHAs of 5 to 12 percent are applied daily to affected skin, they are effective in the treatment of acne vulgaris, ichthyosis (dry, scaly, "fishlike" skin condition) wrinkles, sun-damaged skin, and wound healing. Alphahydroxy acids are also helpful in the treatment of age spots and help to restore skin elasticity. Because AHA therapy is a long-term, maintenance treatment, many individuals must use it indefinitely. For severe or chronic skin conditions, higher concentrations of AHAs can be applied and "peeled" off. This procedure, called a skin peel, must be done by a physician.

Alphahydroxy acids can be either synthetics or natural extractions. Synthetic forms contain 70 percent acid and 30 percent chemical additives, some of which may be irritating. Naturally extracted (ultrapure crystalline grade) AHAs are 100 percent acid and are purified by a process called recrystallization, which makes it pharmaceutical quality. Recrystallization removes harmful byproducts and results in a product that is more gentle to the skin.

Amino Acids (ah-MEEN-oh) are simple natural substances that are the building blocks of proteins. The body uses amino acids for growth, maintenance, and the repair and production of enzymes, hormones, and antibodies. Of the twenty-one amino acids, nine are essential (eight in adults; one, histidine, in infants). This means they are necessary for good health but the body cannot synthesize them, so they must be acquired through diet. The remaining twelve are also necessary, but the body produces them (see box).

Amino acids are available as single supplements or as combination mixtures. Amino acid combinations are often taken by individuals who are bodybuilders or in athletic training. Many medical experts, including Andrew Weil, M.D., believe such supplements are unnecessary, as the majority of people already consume too much protein. Amino acid mixtures can place excess stress on the liver and kidneys and irritate the immune system.

A few of the amino acid supplements, when taken alone,

can be beneficial, though. Phenylalanine comes in three forms: L-, D-, and DL-phenylalanine. (The L and D identify slight differences in molecular structure, and the DL form is a combination of the two other forms.) The L-form is used to build proteins and can help relieve depression, the D-form can relieve chronic pain, and the DL-form is helpful for fighting depression and raising energy levels. L-tyrosine is also helpful for depression. L-lysine may reduce the frequency of attacks of cold sores and fever blisters. People who are recovering from injuries or from surgery may get some help from **arginine**, which helps to improve muscle mass. (Arginine is popular among athletes who want muscle-building effects.)

Amino Acids

ESSENTIAL	NONESSENTIAL	
histidine	cysteine	tyrosine
isoleucine	alanine	arginine
lysine	asparagine	aspartic acid
methionine	glutamic acid	glutamine
phenylalanine	glycine	proline
threonine	serine	taurine
tryptophan		
valine		
leucine		

Amma Massage (AH-mah) "Amma" is the Chinese word for **massage**, and amma as a practice of therapeutic touch is believed to be the oldest form of massage. Although it originated in China, it became synonymous with Japanese massage once it was introduced to Japan.

Amma involves the use of the fingers, elbows, palms, and knees to deliver various massage techniques, including stroking, vibration, kneading, and circular pressure. These massage methods are done on the **tsubos**, or energy points, which are located along the **meridians** and correspond to the **acupoints** used in **acupressure**. Similar to acupressure therapists, those who practice amma believe that stimulation of the energy points promotes the flow of **chi** and allows the body to heal itself.

Amma practitioners work all 140 tsubos of the body in a specific sequence ritual, called *Kata*. This approach ensures that the body's entire energy field is involved. As practitioners work, they also try to form bonds with their clients as they focus their healing thoughts into each tsubo. It is believed that forming these connections improves the desired results.

ALSO SEE massage

Angelica (an-JEL-i-kuh) is a broad term for several herbs in the parsley and carrot family that are used for healing. *Angelica sinensis*, or Chinese angelica, is a popular Chinese herb used to treat gynecological problems. It is also known as *dang-qui* or *tang-kuei* and is related to the European angelica *(Angelica archangelica)*, which was popular in medieval Europe as a protection against witchcraft and illness. American angelica *(Angelica atropurpurea)* is yet another form of this herb. The latter two species are sometimes known as wild celery.

European angelica burst into prominence during the bubonic plague epidemic in 1665 when a monk had a dream in which an angel told him that wild celery was a cure for the disease. The monk renamed the wild celery plant ''angelica,'' and within a few years the British Royal College of Physicians had added the herb to *The King's Excellent Plague Recipe*.

American angelica was already a popular treatment for respiratory conditions among Native Americans when the European settlers came to North America. The new Americans soon found another use for the herb—to induce abortion—and the nineteenth-century American Eclectic physicians prescribed it to their patients who had bronchitis, typhoid, malaria, and heartburn.

Chinese and Indian **Ayurvedic** physicians, who have been using angelica since ancient times, maintain that Chinese angelica is more effective than the European and American species for improving red blood cell counts, stimulating secretion of estrogen, relaxing the uterus, relieving menopausal symptoms, and boosting the immune system. Both the European and American species of angelica are often recommended for stomach pain, heartburn, gas, colds, flu, and fever.

Antioxidants (an-tee-OK-si-dants) are nutrients that attack and eliminate harmful free radicals, highly charged molecules that are believed to be instrumental in the aging process and in contributing to the development of cancer and other diseases. Many different vitamins, minerals, and other nutrients act as antioxidants, and each one has its own specific function in the body and its own free radicals it can eliminate effectively. Some of the most commonly recognized and used antioxidants include vitamin C, vitamin E, beta-carotene, and **selenium**, as well as **flavonoid**-rich supplements such as **pycnogenol**, **green tea**, and **ginkgo**.

Antioxidant supplements are generally taken by individuals who want to counteract the negative effects of free radicals, which are found naturally in the body as well as throughout the environment: in air pollution, tobacco smoke, pesticides, alcoholic beverages, chemotherapeutic agents, and other chemicals. The body may store or use different amounts of antioxidants, depending on its needs at a particular time. Although diet should be the main source of antioxidants, many experts recommend taking a variety of supplements to ensure adequate protection, as the body is in constant need of antioxidant enzymes and nutrients to protect against the damage that is waged continuously by free radicals.

Apis (AY-pis) *(Apis mellifica)* is a homeopathic remedy prepared from the entire honeybee, including the venom. Indications for its use include: sharp, stinging pain, red-

COMMON ANTIOXIDANTS

Beta-carotene: breaks down environmental toxins; boosts the immune system

Vitamin E: protects all cells from free-radical damage; protects vitamins A and C from destruction

Vitamin C: assists in antibody response; stimulates immune system cells; improves the mobility of white blood cells; reduces cancer rates; protects against air pollutants; increases life expectancy; strengthens blood vessel walls; aids in wound healing

Vitamin B1: neutralizes free radicals; counteracts the effects of cigarette smoke and alcohol

Vitamin B2 (riboflavin)**:** keeps the mucosal lining healthy so it can fight off infection

Vitamin B3 (niacinamide)**:** plays a key role in the production of the brain's neurotransmitters

Vitamin B5 (pantothenic acid)**:** works in the brain to produce intercellular energy; also may stimulate cells of the immune system

Vitamin B6: involved in the production of nucleic acid and protein, both of which are required by the immune network

Vitamin B12: needed for maturation of immune system cells

Folic acid: needed for maturation of immune system cells

Zinc: critical cofactor in more than 100 enzymes; stimulates the T-cells, facilitates production of natural killer cells

Copper: boosts functioning of immune system cells

Selenium: slows aging process; protects against chemical hypersensitivity

Coenzyme Q-10: anti-aging and immune-boosting functions; e.g., increases production of antibodies, reduces

> high blood pressure, and improves blood flow and strength of people with heart disease
>
> **Pycnogenol:** helps memory; reduces senility; slows cell mutation that occurs with aging
>
> **Manganese:** helps fight free radical damage

ness, and swelling—all of which develop rapidly. There may be a tightness throughout the abdomen and scant urination, although the urge to urinate may be strong. People who suffer from skin infections, bites, arthritis, sore throat, hives, and eye infections and who are generally fearful, apathetic, irritable, whiny, and restless may benefit the most from apis. Generally, patients feel better in cold settings, whether it be air conditioning, cold fluids, or cold compresses, and worse in hot settings.
ALSO SEE homeopathy

Apitherapy (a-pe-THER-e-pe) is the medicinal use of products from honeybees, such as honey, pollen, propolis, royal jelly, and venom. Bee therapy has been a part of folk medicine for more than 2,000 years. Hippocrates used it to treat arthritis and other painful conditions, and people throughout Europe and Russia have used it for centuries to treat lumbago, rheumatism, and gout.

Injection of bee venom, either through a needle or a direct bee sting, is the primary form of apitherapy. Bee venom relieves inflammatory conditions by stimulating the body's immune system in a circuitous way. When bee venom is introduced into the body, it causes inflammation, which the body combats by producing anti-inflammatory hormones. If bee venom is introduced into an area that is already inflamed, the hormones attack both the venom and the original inflammation and provide relief. Because bee therapy helps the body heal itself, a series of injections or stings are needed to support healing. Bee venom also contains various bactericidal and analgesic components.

Raw honey, the main "product" of bees, is rich in vitamins, minerals, trace elements, and live enzymes. It also has bactericidal, anti-allergic, and anti-inflammatory properties. Both bee pollen and propolis are suspended in honey and impart their benefits to it. Some of the most interesting uses for honey are topical: for wounds, burns, and decubitus ulcers. Its use is believed to accelerate the healing process.

Bee pollen is pollen gathered by bees to which they add their own "special ingredients," which scientists have yet to fully identify. Bee pollen is sometimes called a "complete food" because it contains all the nutrients people need to support life. **Propolis** is the sticky resin that is secreted from the buds and bark of some trees. Bees gather propolis and mix it with wax that is secreted from glands in their abdomens. It has powerful antimicrobial properties and has been called "Russian penicillin" because of its effective use in that country against various fungal and bacterial infections.

Royal jelly is a thick, creamy fluid produced by nurse bees (young bees that feed the larva) during digestion of bee pollen. It is rich in hormones, B vitamins, 20 amino acids, and vitamins A, C, and E. Royal jelly has been credited with stimulating the circulatory system, boosting metabolism, and facilitating gland and cell functioning.

According to the American Apitherapy Society, individuals who use apitherapy report success in treating conditions such as eczema, psoriasis, skin ulcers, laryngitis, herpes simplex, warts, various types of arthritis (rheumatoid, traumatic, psoriatic, juvenile rheumatoid, osteoarthritis, and bursitis), hypertension, atherosclerosis, varicose veins, chronic obstructive pulmonary disease, emphysema, asthma, hearing loss, glaucoma, depression, premenstrual syndrome, menstrual cramps, and decreased blood sugar. (About 2 percent of the population is allergic to bee venom, and in rare cases exposure is fatal.) Since the 1970s, the Chinese have combined bee venom and acupuncture to treat epilepsy, impotency, and other ailments. Veterinarians also use bee venom to treat arthritis in dogs and horses.

Applied Kinesiology (kuh-nee-see-AL-uh-jee) is a two-step, noninvasive scientific approach that combines the principles of body mechanics and anatomy to bring the body back into balance. The approach involves testing the muscles in the body in relation to all body functions to identify any imbalances as well as evaluating lifestyle and prescribing nutritional therapy, emotional support, and bodywork to return the body to harmony. It is often confused with standard kinesiology, which is the study of the mechanical and anatomical principles of human movement.

The birth of applied kinesiology occurred in the early twentieth century when several osteopaths and a chiropractor explored how certain reflex points related to problems in different muscle groups and to the endocrine system. But it wasn't until 1964 that a chiropractor named George Goodheart found that when he applied pressure to certain weak muscles he could restore strength to them. He also became aware of the link between the ancient Chinese concept of **chi**—natural energy flow in the body—and Western medical thought and that he could monitor that energy using muscle tests. He and his colleagues expanded on the initial observations of the early part of the century. The result was applied kinesiology. **Touch for Health** was introduced in the 1970s as a self-help form of applied kinesiology.

Those who practice applied kinesiology—practitioners who are licensed to diagnose, such as medical doctors, chiropractors, dentists, and osteopaths—perform a physical assessment to determine where imbalances are hiding in the body. Once these blockages are identified—be they chemical, structural, or emotional—treatment can begin. Kinesiology can also be used to treat or locate potential "trouble spots" even before symptoms are evident.

Applied kinesiology can help relieve stress, back and neck pain, fatigue, and depression; boost energy levels and stamina; improve breathing, digestion, and concentration; and resolve food intolerance, food sensitivities, acne, headache, and eczema.

ALSO SEE contact reflex analysis; reflexology

Applied Physiology is a system of stress management in which biofeedback and muscle and fascia monitoring are used to identify imbalances in the body and to help correct the stress-producing conditions. It was introduced by George Utt, who worked extensively with **applied kinesiology**, anatomy, **biofeedback**, and various healing techniques before he developed this approach. Applied physiology is based on the concept that specific muscles are linked with various organ and body systems through the **acupuncture/acupressure meridian** system. To locate stress levels in the organs, tissues, meridians, and body systems, applied physiologists monitor a muscle that is in balance—commonly referred to as the "indicator muscle"—while testing various points on the body. Changes that occur in the indicator muscle during this process help identify the energy and stress levels present in affected areas throughout the body. Applied physiologists then use that information to relieve the stress and correct the imbalances through the use of acupressure.

Applied physiology is used to treat people who have polio, muscular dystrophy, and other muscle disorders; it may relieve skin ailments, stress caused by environmental factors, and/or trauma and food allergies.

ALSO SEE applied kinesiology; contact reflex analysis

Arginine (AR-je-neen) is one of the essential **amino acids** in the human body. A primary function of arginine is to produce nitric oxide, which helps the cardiovascular system in several ways: it relaxes the arterial walls, helps reduce spasms in the arteries, and slows down plaque development within the arterial walls. These properties make arginine helpful in people with hypertension, angina, or other types of heart conditions. Arginine is also credited with aiding liver detoxification, retarding tumor growth, maintaining a healthy immune system, generating healthy tissue, and increasing sperm counts in males.

Arginine is found in protein foods and is most prevalent

in spirulina and soybeans. Split peas, lentils, chick-peas, peanuts, tofu, and navy beans also contain significant amounts.

Arnica (AR-nih-kuh) *(Arnica montana)*, also known as leopard's bane, sneezewort, and mountain tobacco, is a plant with a daisylike flower that grows wild in the mountains of western North America, Europe, and Siberia. For centuries it has been used to treat the injuries, aches, and pains of mountain climbers and country folk.

Arnica has gained a reputation among homeopaths and herbalists as being the "first aid treatment of choice" for people who experience physical and emotional shock, pain, bruising, and injuries associated with surgery, accidents, sporting events, dental work, childbirth, and grief. It is also effective for gout, osteoarthritis, sleeplessness caused by overexhaustion, toothache, loss of voice, and bee or wasp stings. Its ability to reduce inflammation and pain is attributed to a chemical compound, lactone helenalin, among others.

In most cases, arnica is applied topically. It is toxic if ingested except in the form of homeopathic tablets, which are too dilute to cause harm. Conditions that warrant internal use include eczema and boils, eyestrain, and fever characterized by a hot head and a cold body. Arnica is effective in children who have whooping cough or who wet the bed because of nightmares.
ALSO SEE homeopathy

Aromatherapy (a-RO-muh-THER-uh-pee) is the use of the **essential oils** of plants for therapeutic purposes, be they medicinal, psychological, or aesthetic. **Essential oils** (or aromatic oils) refer to the fragrant fluid that is extracted from the flowers, root, bark, or resin of plants. These oils are used topically with **massage**, floated in bath water, or inhaled for their therapeutic effects. Depending on the plant from which the oil is derived, its effect may be as an antidepressant, diuretic, antibacterial, or relaxant.

For thousands of years, various civilizations and societies have used fragrances for their ability to help the healing process and to ease stress. Interest in aromatherapy in the United States is a recent development and grew out of the work of a French chemist named Rene-Maurice Gattefosse, who founded a perfumery in France during the 1920s. While he was blending a new perfume, an explosion rocked his laboratory and burned his arm. He plunged his arm into a bowl of lavender oil and quickly experienced relief. When he noticed that his arm was healing much more quickly than burns normally do and without scar tissue, he turned to the study of essential oils and how they can affect health.

Although a scientific basis for the benefits of aromatherapy has yet to be determined definitively, aromatherapists claim essential oils can effectively treat symptoms and conditions such as arthritis, depression, the common cold, sinus infections, stress, menstrual cramps, insomnia, headache, varicose veins, and hiccups. There are two ways essential oils enter and affect the body: through the skin and the nose. During an oiled massage or while soaking in a tub of oils and hot water, the oils penetrate the skin and enter into the tissues and the lymphatic system and may either work at that site or be carried by body fluids throughout the body. For example, if juniper oil, which has diuretic properties, is massaged into an area that is swollen, it can help flush out the fluid.

It is theorized that when essential oils are inhaled, about five million smell-detecting cells activate and the olfactory nerve carries the aroma to the areas of the brain that control hormonal response and emotions. The scent of basil, for example, is believed to help relieve the blues, while **lavender** reportedly can increase awareness while decreasing stress.
ALSO SEE Swedish massage

Art Therapy is the use of painting, sculpting, drawing, or other crafts as a therapeutic form of nonverbal expression. This creative technique has been an established therapeutic method since the early 1970s. It is useful for: individuals who find it difficult to express their emotions, those too young or who are otherwise incapable of verbal expression, people with severe mental problems, and those who have deep-seated issues they cannot express in words.

Art therapy first dawned as a concept in the early 1800s when some individuals involved in the treatment of the mentally ill discussed the validity of exposing this population to the arts. Unfortunately, this idea wasn't put into practice, although the concept stayed alive. Art therapy as a profession was initiated around 1915 by Margaret Naumburg, a teacher who became a psychologist and used art therapy with her patients as part of their treatment. The art therapy movement grew slowly and resulted in the formation of the American Art Therapy Association in 1969.

Art therapists make diagnostic assessments and plan therapy programs based on: their observations of a client's behavior during the creation process, the symbolism in the artwork, which medium and materials the client uses, and any other communication that occurs during a session. Art therapy is often used to treat psychological and behavioral problems, eating disorders, digestive ailments, headaches, and stress-related conditions.

ALSO SEE dance therapy; music therapy

Ashwaganda (ash-wah-GAHN-dah) *(Withania somnifera)*, also known as Ayurvedic winter cherry, is an **Ayurvedic** herb that grows in India. It has a reputation as an aphrodisiac and has traditionally been used to help prevent male sterility and other sexual problems.

Today as in the past, the roots, berries, and leaves of ashwaganda are used to prepare tinctures and powders used to make infusions and decoctions. The oral remedies can be used to help restore muscular strength and to treat multiple sclerosis, rheumatism, indigestion, and heart disease. The medicated oil, which consists of ashwaganda leaves, castor oil, and water, can be applied to inflammations, sores, and swelling, while a compress soaked in an infusion is effective against ringworm.

Aston Patterning is a type of movement therapy that integrates various soft-tissue **bodywork** techniques, education regarding movement patterns, and environmental modifications as a way to regain natural ease of movement, grace, coordination, and resilience, and to ease pain. It is the brainchild of Judith Aston, who was led to develop this system as a result, in early years, of an interest in movement and dance and, in later years, personal medical problems. When automobile accidents left this dance teacher with severe neck and back injuries, she sought alternatives to surgery and underwent **rolfing** treatments. Aston was so impressed with the results that she studied rolfing with Dr. Ida Rolf and eventually developed her own philosophy and system of bodywork.

According to Aston, people develop "patterns" of movement and posture based on their bodies' histories of trauma, physical activity, the amount of stress they encounter, and their mental attitudes. These patterns manifest in different areas of the body and are a reflection of the tension the body holds. Aston patterning helps people make positive changes and correct physical problems through education, often by videotaping a person's movements to determine which habits are contributing to the problem; gentle massage; and environmental consultation and adjustments, which includes an evaluation of the person's home and work places, identification of any objects that may be contributing to the problem, and steps to modify those things earmarked as such.

Aston patterning is often used by dancers and athletes as well as individuals seeking relief from back and neck pain, postural problems, headache, and other manifestations of chronic physical and mental stress.

Astragalus (a-STRAG-uh-lus) (*Astragalus membranaceas*) is an herb that grows in northeastern China. It is commonly used in **Chinese medicine**, where it is usually called *huang chi*. The Chinese have revered this herb for thousands of years for its ability to treat anemia, night sweats, weakness, lack of vitality, and poor appetite.

Today, astragalus is valued as a tonic, diuretic, stimulant, and antibacterial agent. Medical researchers in China have shown astragalus to increase levels of antibodies, promote the healing of damaged tissues, eliminate toxins, and stabilize blood pressure. Chinese herbalists consider this herb to be one of the best immune-boosting agents available. To increase its immune-boosting abilities and its ability to harmonize function of the internal organs, astragalus is often processed with honey and it can be purchased in this form. Western herbalists attribute astragalus's healing abilities to its polysaccharides (complex carbohydrates).

Aura (AW-ra) is an energy or a magnetic field that is said to surround all people, plants, and animals. It radiates out and away from the body, much like a halo, and may be of various colors. Each color—there are nine main colors (black/gray, blue, green, indigo, orange, red, yellow, violet, and white)—reportedly reveals a person's physical, mental, emotional, and spiritual states, or the general condition of a plant or animal. Auras have been depicted in many cultures: as golden halos in early Christian artwork, and as areas of glowing or vibrating light in aboriginal paintings, on Native American totem poles, and in Eastern sculpture.

Some people have been reported to have the ability to detect auras by touch, clairvoyance, or intuition. Touch is the most common way healers discern energy fields, and the most popular way is to use their hands to "scan" areas of an individual's body. As healers pass their hands over the body of a client, they report feelings of heat, cold, tingling, pain, throbbing, and other sensations which indicate areas where the individual is experiencing pain, disease, or other problems. Some healers say they can see and interpret auras, while others "sense" their presence by looking at a photograph. A process called **Kirlian photography**, developed by Russian engineer Semyon Kirlian, is said to reveal auras.

Auricular Therapy (aw-RIK-u-luhr) involves treating acupuncture points on the external ear. It has been practiced for more than 1,000 years and has been the subject of research and development in France and China in recent years. This **acupuncture** technique has gained considerable recognition for: its effectiveness in treating allergic conditions, drug and alcohol addictions, headache, migraine, sinus problems, respiratory disorders, gastrointestinal disorders, and for pain control, especially in terminal illness.

Practitioners need to be highly trained to accurately choose from the more than 120 points that can be treated on each ear. These points mirror the entire human body, thus auricular therapy can be used to treat the same ailments as those treated using full-body acupuncture. Once the needles have been placed, they may be kept in for approximately 15 minutes or held in place with an adhesive patch for several days, depending on the condition being treated. Experts believe auricular therapy, like full-body acupuncture, works neuroelectrically. That is, the inserted needles connect with and stimulate the nerves and trigger the release of the body's natural painkillers, called endorphins. Like acupuncture needles that are placed elsewhere on the body, the needles used in auricular therapy may be manipulated or electrically stimulated as needed.
ALSO SEE acupuncture

Autogenic Training (aw-toe-JEN-ik) is a form of self-hypnosis in which people get into a relaxed, passive state of mind and complete a series of exercises and suggestions designed to teach them how to deal with the ways their bodies react to stress. Dr. Johannes Schultz, who developed autogenic training in 1929, found that once people put themselves into altered states of awareness, they can achieve relief from stress and tension, and often any associated physical conditions, by silently completing a series of six mental exercises that focus on the following goals: relaxing the legs and arms, regulating the heartbeat, achieving a natural breathing pattern, cooling the forehead, warming the abdomen, and relieving suppressed negative emotions (which involves the use of "intentional" exercises). The six mental exercises are designed to regulate blood flow, improve energy levels, promote self-healing through deep relaxation, and promote well-being and health; the intentional exercises, as stated, help relieve suppressed emotions.

Autogenic training is a holistic technique—it treats the whole person rather than specific symptoms. Because it treats the entire body, many conditions respond well to autogenic training, such as: headache, insomnia, premenstrual syndrome, high blood pressure, asthma, eczema, muscle pain, diabetes, thyroid disorders, and diarrhea.

ALSO SEE hypnotherapy

Ayurvedic Medicine (ah-yoor-VAY-dik) is a healing system that originated in India more than 5,000 years ago. Historical documentation of Ayurveda has been found in ancient books of wisdom known as the Vedas, which list, among other things, remedies and techniques to deal with specific ailments such as: gallstones, high blood pressure, peptic ulcers, bronchitis, and acne.

A primary goal of Ayurveda—which loosely translated from Sanskrit means "life" *(ayu)* "knowledge" *(veda)*—is to guide individuals in their food choices and lifestyle so they can live in harmony and balance their bodies, minds, and spirits with external forces. To achieve these goals, Ayurveda adheres to several basic concepts.

Key to Ayurveda is the belief in the mind-body connection and that the mind and body communicate with one another at all times. Ayurveda also teaches that everyone embodies an energy or "soul" that existed before we had our physical bodies. Another belief is that all physical objects, including people, animals, and plants, are composed of microscopic particles that are in constant motion. When these particles are in chaos or flow abnormally, disease is the result.

In order to restore harmony, or normal particle flow, to a body with disease, the Ayurvedic method is to use the mind, along with any one or more of the five senses, to affect the particles. There is a growing body of evidence that thoughts and emotions can influence and even control bodily functions (see **biofeedback**, for example). Thus you can use your mind and body together to regulate your physical and emotional being. Examples of how you can use your senses to heal include: taking herbs or modifying your

---

AYURVEDIC DOSHAS

Every individual has either a clearly dominant dosha or some combination of any two or all three. General characteristics of the three individual doshas are explained briefly below, along with the diseases most often associated with each mind-body type.

Vata people tend to have a lot of energy and enthusiasm. They need to keep active to stay in balance. When they lack something constructive to do, they tend to fidget or waste energy. Vata conditions: intestinal gas, sciatica, arthritis, paralysis, neuralgia, low back pain, and nervous system disease.

Pitta people are transformers: they like to take a situation and change it into something else. Often they are competitive and possess anger, aggressiveness, or irritability. Pitta conditions: gastritis, peptic ulcer, hyperacidity, skin disorders, liver and bile disorders, and inflammatory diseases such as rheumatoid arthritis.

Kapha people are often heavier, more solid and tranquil, and slower moving than people in the other doshas. Kapha conditions include bronchitis, sinusitis, lung congestion, and tonsillitis.

diet (taste); inhalation of specific aromas (smell; see **aromatherapy**); **massage** (touch); and **sound therapy**, which can stimulate chemicals in the body (hearing; see **music therapy**).

In Ayurveda, everyone is viewed as being composed of five main elements—space, air, fire, water, and earth—with each person being a unique combination of these elements. There are three primary mind-body types, or doshas, that result from combining the five elements: vata, kapha, and pitta (see box). If you visit an Ayurvedic physician, she or he may prescribe herbal remedies, specific foods, or perhaps meditation or massage, based on your particular dosha. Thus your treatment plan will be specially tailored to your unique mind-body state.

Bach Flower Remedies (batch) involve ingestion of the "essences" of certain flowers as a way to overcome negative emotions, which, according to the developer of this modality, Edward Bach, M.D., are responsible for illness. Bach remedies are designed to restore emotional balance, a sense of calm, and physical well-being.

Flower essences are prepared by floating the fresh blossoms of selected plants in containers of spring water that are left in sunlight on a cloudless day. According to Dr. Bach (1886-1936), this allows the essence, or inherent energy, of the flowers to enter the water and "potentize" it. Brandy is added to the potentized water to preserve it, and the completed remedy is stored in a dark glass bottle.

A remedy is taken by placing a few drops of the essence into a little bit of mineral water and sipping the mixture.

Bach and homeopathic remedies are similar in that they both are purported to work at the body's physical and psychological energy levels, rather than chemically, as do herbal remedies. Flower remedies are reportedly effective in treating nervous disorders, depression, mood swings, fear, exhaustion, anxiety, asthma, premenstrual tension, eczema, and psoriasis. They are also useful when applied topically for burns, bites, and bruises.

Bach identified 38 flowers that offer relief for specific types of negative feelings and emotions. For example, holly is used for jealousy, anger, revenge, and suspicion; sweet chestnut is for overwhelming desolation. He developed a combination remedy called Rescue Remedy (cherry plum, clematis, impatiens, star of Bethlehem, and rock rose), which he believed relieves the effects of shock, trauma, or other stressful situations. This and other Bach remedies are available through health food stores, natural food stores, and mail order outlets. A renewed interest in **flower remedies** in the 1970s prompted research into additional remedies and the introduction of some new essences.
ALSO SEE homeopathy

Bates Method of Vision Training is a natural, holistic program of physical and mental exercises designed to treat vision problems that do not have an organic cause. It was developed by William Horatio Bates, M.D. (1881-1931), an ophthalmologist whose research led him to find that many vision defects are caused by weakness of the six intrinsic eye muscles, which in turn prevents the lens from focusing correctly. The weakness, he reported, is caused by eyestrain and nervous tension, and once these factors are eliminated, the eye muscles can focus optimally. He then developed a series of relaxation and eye exercises that relieve tension and stress and strengthen the eye muscles.

The Bates Method is useful for correcting hazy vision, tired eyes, and squint (inward or outward turning of the eye, normally caused by damage to the eye muscles), and may help prevent some people from needing glasses to correct near- or farsightedness. It does not cure glaucoma or cataracts but does strengthen the eye muscles.

Bee Pollen consists of the pollen gathered by bees, plus special, as-yet-unidentified ingredients added by the bees. This "ambrosia of the gods" has been touted as a source of perpetual youth and health since ancient times. The ancient Egyptians, Hebrews, Orientals, and South American natives used a combination of bee pollen and honey to treat burns, wounds, and boils. In several Asian cultures, this same mixture is added to vegetable or fruit juice and used as a health drink.

Bee pollen is considered to be a complete food because it contains 22 amino acids, including all the essential ones; 27 minerals, including calcium, iron, and magnesium; enzymes, which improve metabolism and digestion; and all vitamins, including B12. Research conducted by the U.S. Department of Agriculture has suggested that bee pollen has anticancer properties. Bee pollen is used to treat allergies, boost the immune system to help it fight environmental toxins and viral infections, normalize weight, relieve fatigue, improve concentration, increase sexual potency, and relieve headache. There is also anecdotal evidence that bee pollen is effective in treating attention deficit disorder.

Bee pollen is available in capsules and can be taken as a supplement or added to foods such as fruit and vegetable juices, soups, rice, and puddings. Do not heat or cook bee pollen, however, as intense heat destroys its nutrients. ALSO SEE apitherapy; royal jelly

Belladonna *(Atropa belladonna)*, which means "beautiful woman," is one of the most widely used homeopathic remedies. It is commonly known as deadly nightshade and is aptly named, as every part of the plant is poisonous. When used in homeopathic remedies, however, it should be safe because either none or only a minute amount of the plant is in the remedy.

Belladonna grows throughout Europe and has been a part

of European culture for centuries. It was reportedly used in witchcraft during the Middle Ages, and Italian women used belladonna as an eyedrop to make their pupils dilate and their eyes more beautiful. Dr. Samuel Hahnemann, the father of **homeopathy**, added the plant to his homeopathic remedies in 1799 and used it to treat scarlet fever.

Today, belladonna is used to treat conditions that involve inflammation, and complaints that come on suddenly; for example, flu, tonsillitis, sore throat, high fever accompanied by dilated eyes, earache, teething, swollen joints, menstrual cramps, abdominal pain, pounding headache, seizures, labor pain, cystitis, nephritis (inflamed kidneys), restless sleep, and any condition that includes the following symptoms: bright red tongue; throbbing pain; pale lips and mouth; red, hot face; dry, flushed skin; cold hands and feet; and extreme sensitivity to light, pressure, touch, noise, and movement. Belladonna has also been given to children to reduce fever and to ease teething pain.

Homeopathic experts and some naturopaths believe belladonna derives some of its healing properties from atropine and hyoscine, two alkaloids used in conventional medicine to treat vertigo, nausea, and spasms.

Benjamin System of Muscular Therapy

Benjamin System of Muscular Therapy, developed in 1967, is a program that combines education and treatment; both are designed to eliminate chronic muscle tension and promote overall physical health. The creation of this system represents the efforts of Ben E. Benjamin, Ph.D., who studied and drew from the work of several individuals and their techniques, including F.M. Alexander and the **Alexander Technique** and English orthopedist James Cyriax.

The Benjamin System consists of tension-relieving exercises, deep massage treatments, body-care techniques, and body alignment movements. This program reportedly helps to eliminate chronic muscle tension, specifically mechanical tension that is the result of poor posture, injuries, surgery, improper movement and body alignment, and environmental stressors. Dr. Benjamin outlined seven hundred specific movements that not only promote relaxation and stress reduction, but also may benefit those with sports injuries and other musculoskeletal problems.

Bilberry *(Vaccinium myrtillus)* is a blue-black berry that grows on a shrub found mostly in Europe. It is most notably used to treat and prevent vision problems, as it is rich in certain **flavonoids** that are known to aid eyesight.

Bilberry's medicinal value was found serendipitously when it was noted that British Royal Air Force pilots during World War II had excellent night vision. All of these pilots were eating bilberry jam before their night missions. Spurred by these reports, scientists conducted tests on the berries and discovered they contain vision-enhancing flavonoids called anthocyanosides. These substances significantly increase the ability of the eye to adjust to the dark, and also appear to be helpful in the temporary relief of chronic eye fatigue and day blindness. Routine consumption of bilberry may help prevent glaucoma and cataracts, and it may help slow the progression of macular degeneration. As a preventive measure, bilberry is helpful for people who do much close work, night drivers, students, and those who work on computer monitors. It is available in capsule and extract forms.

Biochemic Tissue Salts Therapy is a self-help treatment that is based on the theory that cells need to maintain a specific balance of natural mineral salts to stay healthy. When one or more mineral salts is deficient in the body, an imbalance occurs and may lead to disease and illness. Biochemic Tissue Salts Therapy resolves those deficiencies and facilitates the body's return to balance.

W.H. Schuessler, the German homeopath who developed this supplemental therapeutic approach in the 1870s, identified 12 tissue salts and their effects. Today, Biochemic Tissue Salts are usually prescribed by naturopaths, homeopaths, and herbalists to complement other natural therapies. The salts are prepared in the same way as homeopathic remedies and are believed not to have any adverse effects. Which mineral salt is prescribed depends on the presenting condition or symptoms.

Many disorders reportedly respond to mineral salts therapy, including: acidity, acne, arthritis, asthma, blisters and boils, bronchitis, chicken pox, circulation disorders, colds and flu, coughs, cramps, cystitis, fever, gout, hay fever, heartburn, indigestion, low-back pain, migraines, mumps, nausea and vomiting, nerve disorders, neuralgia, panic attacks, prostate problems, sciatica, vaginitis, and wheezing. Mineral salts can be purchased at pharmacies and health food stores.
ALSO SEE homeopathy

Biodynamic Massage is an offshoot of **bioenergetics** and is an integration of **massage** and exercise designed to release emotional tension. It was developed by a Norwegian therapist, Gerda Boyesen. During a biodynamic massage session, clients are taught how to "get in touch with" and experience energy as it flows through them. Making this connection can bring up repressed feelings and memories, both negative and positive, and have a freeing effect. As such, biodynamic massage relieves emotional tension as well as physical symptoms and conditions associated with chronic, repressed emotional tension, such as headache, neck and back pain, digestive problems, insomnia, and asthma.
ALSO SEE energy therapies

Bioenergetics is a type of psychotherapy in which individuals free blocked energy—manifested as muscle tension—using breathing techniques, psychotherapy, active exercises (e.g., aerobic activities such as walking and swimming), and **bodywork**. It was developed by Alexander Lowen and John Pierrakos and is based on the work of Wilhelm Reich (1897-1957), a psychiatrist who believed that tensing the muscles is the body's way of "armoring" itself against emotional and mental pain. This pain begins to accumulate at birth, builds over time, and becomes chronic. It remains trapped in the body and affects overall health, movement, and breathing and has negative effects on emotional well-being.

Therapists trained in bioenergetics work with clients to achieve three specific goals: (1) to empower individuals to understand how personality affects the body; (2) to improve all aspects of the personality by releasing repressed muscular tension; and (3) to increase people's ability to experience personal growth and pleasure by resolving attitudes developed as a result of held tensions, which interfere with the body's natural, rhythmic movements. To achieve these goals, bioenergetics utilizes breathing exercises, massage, physical exercises (developed by Lowen to relieve chronically tense muscles), and psychological techniques such as psychodrama, all of which allow people to become aware of repressed traumas, release them, and come to a resolution.

Treatment is highly individualized, and not everyone seeks or gets relief from physical problems. Bioenergetics can be helpful, however, in relieving asthma, migraine, headache, ulcers, sleep disorders, irritable bowel syndrome, and stress.

ALSO SEE biodynamic massage; Reichian therapy

Biofeedback is a procedure whereby people can use special instruments, learned techniques, or both, to receive information *from* the body about what is happening *in* the body. These methods help amplify the subtle physiological messages the body gives out, which in turn allows people to regulate or control certain internal functions—for example, breathing rate, blood circulation to specific parts of the body, and muscle contractions—that are causing pain or discomfort.

Biofeedback means "living" *(bio)* feedback. The brain constantly sends out signals and then it responds to those signals. Some signals are obvious—hunger pangs are one example. Usually, however, a response occurs without the person being aware of it. If you are frightened, for example, your body automatically sends a shot of adrenaline into your system; if you are experiencing a great deal of stress, you may grind your teeth while you sleep. Once you learn biofeedback, you can take control of the mechanisms that cause you pain or anxiety, or are associated with a medical condition such as high blood pressure.

The most common form of biofeedback is electromyographic biofeedback, in which a sensor is attached to the skin over the painful or tense area. The sensor transmits back to a recording device the amount of electrical activity in that location. You can use this feedback to determine which muscles need to relax, and watch your progress on a gauge or other measuring instrument on the recording device. Many people use **visualization therapy** or **imagery** techniques to help them during biofeedback sessions.

In thermal biofeedback, a sensor reveals skin temperature, which is an indication of blood flow changes. Temperature biofeedback can help you learn to increase blood circulation in your hands and feet, an important goal if you suffer with migraine headache, hypertension, anxiety, or Raynaud's disease. Other types of biofeedback include electrodermal (measures subtle changes in perspiration), finger pulse (measures heart rate and force), and monitoring breathing patterns (measures breath rate, rhythm, volume, and location).

Biofeedback therapy was developed in the United States in the 1970s. Since then it has gained acceptance for use in treating conditions such as headache and migraine, muscle tension, chronic pain, incontinence, hypertension, anxiety, asthma, cerebal palsy, constipation, diabetes, teeth grinding, and Raynaud's disease.
ALSO SEE imagery; visualization therapy

Bio-Magnetic Touch Healing is a therapeutic healing technique in which feather-light touch is used to reduce stress, eliminate pain, and provide other curative effects. It is a self-healing method as well as one that can be done for others, and it complements both conventional and natural healing techniques. In just a few hours anyone, regardless of age or professional background, can learn how to do bio-magnetic touch healing.

Like other touch therapies, no one has been able to document scientifically how or why it works. According to certified bio-magnetic touch therapists, the body's own natural healing processes are activated by the light, subtle touch applied to a specific combination of points on the body. With each repeat treatment, healing progresses and symptoms or ailments resolve themselves. Each treatment also leaves the body in a better-balanced, more harmonious state.

Bio-magnetic touch healing is gaining popularity among nurses and other health care professionals who find that it complements their routine care and that its gentle, noninvasive nature makes it agreeable to patients in most any situation.

Black Cohosh (KO-hosh) *(Cimicifuga racemosa)* is a member of the buttercup and peony family of plants, and an herb that has been used for centuries to treat gynecological problems. It is known for its estrogen-like effects and its effect on blood pressure.

The Algonquian tribe of the northeastern United States named this herb for the characteristics of its roots: black for the color and *cohosh* for its texture, "rough." These Native Americans used black cohosh primarily to treat gynecological problems and to help in childbirth. Other uses included treatment of sore throat, arthritis, fatigue, and snakebite. The colonists quickly followed suit and prescribed it for menstrual cramps, skin rashes, fever, insomnia, and malaria. Today it is prescribed by homeopaths and herbalists primarily for menstrual discomfort, pain of childbirth, as a diuretic, and to help clear mucus from the respiratory tract. It is also indicated for use in managing prostate cancer and reducing high blood pressure.

Body Logic is a system of structural therapy that helps people realign the body through the use of traction and rotation of the joints. It is called "body logic" because, as its developer Yamuna Zake explains, the technique allows the body to use "its instinctive knowledge of where it needs to release when given the opportunity."

Body Logic is based on the premise that the muscles have memory, and once muscles that have been held in painful, uncomfortable, or otherwise negative positions are placed in noncontracted postures, they will "remember" the good feeling and correct themselves. Body Logic practitioners use their own bodies for leverage and stretch the client's joints, allowing the muscles to release from where they attach to the bone. After traction, practitioners rotate the joints. Both of these procedures help to realign the body, improve blood circulation, improve flexibility, and increase energy level. Body Logic practitioners are taught to be aware of the body's energy flow and to work with the **chakras**.

Body Logic can benefit people of all ages and relieve the pain associated with headache and migraine, chronic back pain, arthritis, herniated discs, and hunchback curve. Dancers and athletes find this therapy especially helpful for improving movement and for recovering from injuries. Body Logic therapists also claim it to be effective in treating people with epilepsy, stroke, and cerebral palsy.

Body-Mind Centering is a therapeutic movement approach designed to release the stress, tension, fears, pains, and misguided perceptions that prevent people from functioning optimally. People who experience Body-Mind Centering (BMC) learn to increase their awareness of themselves and open up to new options in how to think and feel with greater physical, emotional, and mental freedom.

Body-Mind Centering was created by Bonnie Bainbridge Cohen, whose parents worked for the Ringling Brothers and Barnum & Bailey Circus. Cohen's exposure to a wide variety of performers and her subsequent studies in dance and **dance therapy, yoga, craniosacral therapy, zero balancing, Zen**, and occupational therapy led her to develop her own system of movement therapy. The focus of BMC sessions, according to Cohen, is to allow each individual to become fully aware of his or her own body and each system in it and to initiate movement and action from that awareness. The movements and exercises are designed to increase participants' sensory awareness of their muscles, nerves, organs, skin, fluids, glands, ligaments, and fascia. Cohen explains that everyone has the ability to sense tissues and organs and to move and change them, just as they can sense, move, and change the positions of hands and feet.

Cohen also identified sixteen basic patterns of movement which she says all people progress through, from birth to adulthood. Each subsequent pattern overlaps and depends in some way on the one before it. Therefore, any pattern that is not fully developed can lead to movement and postural problems as life progresses. These underdeveloped patterns can also give rise to problems with perception, memory, creativity, self-esteem, and sociability. Body-Mind Centering allows individuals to create new patterns or repattern old ones.

Each BMC session is tailored to the client's specific needs. Practitioners may use guided **imagery**, movement, hands-on **bodywork**, music, dialogue, or props such as large balls to gently help participants increase sensory awareness. People of all ages can benefit from BMC.

Bodywork is a generic term used to refer to the ever-growing field of massage and other forms of manipulative therapies. By the mid-1990s, more than eighty different varieties of bodywork had been identified. Although each type of bodywork has its own unique philosophy and/or theoretic principles, they all share several basic concepts and benefits. Bodywork can: improve blood circulation, which benefits nearly all health problems; stimulate the lymphatic system; release chronic muscle tension; help restore healthy integration of the body's structure and its functions, which allows all organ systems to operate optimally; promote the reciprocal relationship between mind and body; reduce stress; and encourage energy flow, which promotes healing.

Generally, bodywork helps any health condition that can benefit from improved blood circulation and tension relief. Bodywork tends to complement most other medical therapies and is often used as an enhancement to conventional treatments of backache, constipation, diabetes, muscle pain, and stiff joints, for example.

ALSO SEE massage; specific bodywork and massage therapies by name

Boneset *(Eupatorium perfoliatum)*, also known as feverwort, is an herb used both in **homeopathy** and **herbal medicine**. Its most common use is for relief of symptoms associated with the common cold, flu, and chills. It is also helpful in reducing the aching pain characteristic to rheumatism, especially in the back and limbs.

When prescribed as a homeopathic remedy, symptoms that indicate its use include a cough that is worse at night, sore eyeballs, hoarseness, and an aversion to being touched. As an herbal remedy, it acts as a relaxing agent to the liver and stomach and has a mild laxative effect, and is effective in treating colds and flu, particularly for relieving the aches and pains that accompany fever. It is also used for treating arthritis and rheumatism.

Bowen Technique is a form of bodywork in which therapists administer a series of vibrational movements over the muscles, connective tissue, and tendons to facilitate healing of various musculoskeletal problems. It was introduced by Tom Bowen, an industrial chemist in Australia, in 1974. Since his death in 1982, two of his colleagues, Oswald and Elaine Rentsch, have taught the Bowen Technique around the world.

Bowen was able to recognize minute muscle tensions and used that ability to develop a system of movements to counteract specific body conditions. The Bowen Technique consists of three or four vibrational movements applied to specific points on the body, followed by a rest of two to ten minutes before the next sequence of movements is performed. According to Bowen, this rest period allows the body to "process" each treatment. Back and neck pain, sports injuries, and most musculoskeletal pain respond well to the Bowen Technique.

Breathing Therapies include techniques that help people to focus on and be conscious of their breathing as a way to improve overall energy, boost the immune system, overcome respiratory problems, and reduce tension.

Being conscious of your breathing is of vital importance to many experts in both natural and conventional medicines. From the yogis of India to practicing M.D.s in the United States, the virtues of breathing therapy are being taught by an increasing number of people associated with the healing arts.

Most people don't think about breathing until they have a specific reason to be concerned; for example, they may develop respiratory problems or become short of breath when they overexert themselves. People who have chronic conditions such as asthma or emphysema are much more aware of their breathing. Breathing exercises can benefit anyone, regardless of his or her current state of health, and they can be done anywhere with no need for equipment or preparation.

Breathing is the most effective and efficient way to purify and revitalize the body. Shallow chest breathing, which is the way most adults breathe, allows the body to operate at a minimum level, whereas full, deep breathing sends more healing oxygen and energy to all cells of the body. Three common breathing exercises include deep breathing, hara breathing, and diaphragmatic breathing. In deep breathing, the breath moves deep into the abdomen and the belly rises, then the breath moves up into the diaphragm and upper lungs. In hara breathing, you concentrate on an acupoint that is three fingers' width below the navel as you breathe deep into your belly and feel your lower abdomen rise and fall. In diaphragmatic breathing, you concentrate on allowing the diaphragm, and not the chest, to move air in and out of the lungs. Diaphragmatic breathing is more efficient and relaxing than chest breathing.

Breathing exercises are at the center of many Eastern disciplines and are included as a part of other complementary therapies. During **visualization**, for example, some people find that imagining their breath as healing energy relieves pain or tension. **Yoga**, **meditation**, and other relaxation techniques utilize breathing exercises as part of their healing methods.

ALSO SEE qigong; visualization therapy

Breema Bodywork

is a body therapy that originated among the peoples of Iran and Afghanistan and was brought to the United States by a native villager. It is similar to many other bodywork systems, especially **Thai massage** and **shiatsu**.

Breema bodywork is based on the principle that the body has three energy centers—mind, feelings, and physical body. When there is an imbalance among these three centers, illness results. The movements and postures used in Breema are designed to stimulate the body's self-healing processes, correct any imbalance or weakness, bring clarity to the mind, and invigorate the emotions.

Practitioners trained in Breema bodywork move their client's body in various sequences, from gentle to vigorous, while the client sits or lies on the floor. They also use their palms, feet, forearms, and knees to apply pressure at different sites on the body, although they do not necessarily adhere to the Chinese or Japanese concept of **meridians** or **acupoints**. This portion of the hands-on therapy usually consists of firm but gentle pressure, holds, stretches, bends, and brushes. For those who wish to try Breema on their own, there is a group of exercises called "Self-Breema."

The hundreds of different movement sequences and massage techniques used by Breema practitioners help balance the flow of energy through the body, release stress and tension, increase flexibility and vitality, and improve overall well-being.

Bromelain (BRO-muh-luhn) is an enzyme present in pineapple that assists in the digestion of protein and helps treat diarrhea caused by digestive enzyme deficiency. It also reportedly helps fight cancer, reduce inflammation, and improve blood circulation. Individuals who suffer with sports injuries may take bromelain to help reduce bruising and swelling, relieve pain, and facilitate wound healing.

When purchased as a supplement, bromelain is sometimes combined with papain, an enzyme that comes from unripe papayas. Papain is used in meat tenderizers, and many experts recommend avoiding bromelain supplements that contain this ingredient.

Bryonia (bri-OH-nee-ah) *(Bryonia alba)*, or wild hops, is a member of the gourd family. A homeopathic remedy is made from the root of this vine, which grows in Europe and England. It was one of the first remedies used by Dr. Samuel Hahnemann, the founder of **homeopathy**.

Bryonia is a slow-acting remedy, and it is indicated for complaints that come on slowly and worsen with even the slightest movement. Headache accompanies nearly all other complaints treatable with bryonia, which may include chest pain and coughing, stitching-type pains, very dry mucous membranes, great thirst for cold water, nausea and vomiting, extreme irritability, sluggish mental state, and constipation with dry, hard stools. Symptoms are worse in stuffy rooms and heat, and better when pressure is applied to the painful area and when lying on the painful sites.

The personality profile most suited for bryonia treatment includes individuals who are methodical, calculating, worried about their inability to control their future, easily irritated or angered, and both physically and mentally sluggish. Often they prefer to be left alone when ill. Physically they are above average weight and of dark hair and complexion. Bryonia's therapeutic effects on fibrous tissues, nerve coatings, and other inflamed areas make it effective in individuals with rheumatism.

Calendula (kuh-LEND-you-luh) *(Calendula officinalis)* is a remedy considered one of the staples in a **homeopathy** first aid kit. Several over-the-counter lotions and creams contain calendula. This homeopathic remedy is prepared from the common marigold, and the entire plant is utilized. Calendula is most valued for its anti-inflammatory and antimicrobial properties and is effective in keeping wounds clean and promoting the healing of cuts, burns, and shallow wounds. It should not be used for puncture or deep wounds because it promotes such rapid healing that it may trap infection inside the wound. Other indications include use as a mouthwash to stop bleeding after tooth extraction, and application of the cream to the genital area after childbirth. Because calendula is used primarily as a first aid remedy, no extensive psychological profile has been established for it. Generally, anyone who has a minor injury or wound can benefit from the remedy.

Herbalists also use calendula for many of the same indications as do homeopaths, as well as a few additional ones, including indigestion, gastric ulcers, and earaches. Calendula's healing powers appear to come from its primary component, terpenes, which are compounds that consist of essential oils, fragrances, and flavors.

Capsaicin (cap-SAY-eh-suhn) is the pungent ingredient in **cayenne** (chili peppers) that is effective in reducing various types of pain, including arthritis, peptic ulcers, mouth sores, skin irritations, and neuralgia. The addition of chili peppers to the diet can help relieve the pain associated with these conditions. Several ointments containing capsaicin are available and are effective against shingles (herpes zoster), pain associated with surgical procedures, and cluster headache.

Carbo Vegetabilis (KAR-boh vej-uh-tah-BIL-us) is a homeopathic remedy that is derived from the charcoal of beech, birch, or poplar woods. This remedy is commonly used to treat digestive problems, including bloating and belching. Generally, carbo vegetabilis is effective in individuals who have poor circulation to the hands and feet caused by diabetes or arteriosclerosis; are mentally sluggish and have patchy memory; have cravings for sweets, salty foods, and coffee; experience dry mouth in the morning; and are lazy, listless, and disinterested in life. Elderly people who have a weak and sluggish constitution usually respond well to carbo vegetabilis.
ALSO SEE homeopathy

Carnitine (KAR-nuh-teen) is a vitamin-like substance that promotes the breakdown and transportation of fatty acids, which is essential for the production of cell energy. It is synthesized from the amino acid **lysine** in the liver, brain, and kidneys and needs sufficient levels of vitamin C and iron in order to perform its functions. Healthy human hearts store extra carnitine, but individuals who do not pump enough oxygen into their hearts experience carnitine deficiencies. Supplementation with carnitine can help people with heart disease (including congestive heart failure, cardial myopathies, cardial enlargement, and familial endocardial fibroelastosis), as well as increase good cholesterol levels (high-density lipoprotein, HDL) and decrease bad cholesterol (low-density lipoprotein, LDL) and triglyceride levels.

Fruits, vegetables, and grains have little or no carnitine;

however, the body can manufacture carnitine from lysine, which is abundant in legumes.

Carotenoids (kuh-ROT-uh-noydz) are a class of pigments synthesized by plants that provide the reds, oranges, yellows, and other colors of fruits and vegetables. In green plants, carotenoids are masked by chlorophyll.

Of the approximately 600 carotenoids that are known to exist, only about 20 have been identified as being of significant nutritional value to humans. Foods that contain beneficial carotenoids include tomatoes, orange juice, carrots, and corn. Lycopene, a carotenoid that is in tomatoes, is known to help fight prostate cancer. Alpha- and beta-carotenes are the **antioxidant** carotenoids in carrots, and lutein and zeoxanthin are found in orange juice and corn, and aid vision.

All carotenoids, however, are believed to be valuable antioxidants. They appear to have anticarcinogenic activity in that they prevent the formation of carcinogens that cause tumors. Carotenoids also reduce the amount of free-radical damage to the cells, which in turn inhibits the development and growth of cancers.

Cat's Claw (*Uncaria tomentosa*), also referred to as "uña de gato," is an herb that grows in the South American rainforests. It has been used for centuries for medicinal purposes by the native tribes of the Amazon rainforest.

Cat's claw has been analyzed and found to consist of several alkaloids and phytochemicals that have significant anti-inflammatory effects, which has led to its use in patients with arthritis. Its ability to boost the immune system has been traced to six alkaloids that reside in the inner bark of the plant. Cat's claw also reduces blood pressure, lowers heart rate, promotes blood circulation, and relaxes blood vessels. When buying cat's claw, look for *Uncaria tomentosa*. A close cousin, *Uncaria guianesis*, has similar benefits but lacks immune system advantages.

Cayenne (KY-en) *(Capsicum frutescens)*, also known as hot pepper, cayenne chili pepper, and several other names, has been prized in Asia since ancient times for its culinary value. It was unknown in Europe until Columbus brought it back from the New World, and it soon was noted for its ability to "help digestion, provoke urine, relieve toothache, . . . comfort a cold stomach, expel the stone from the kidney, and take away dimness of sight," according to English herbalist Nicholas Culpeper. Unknown to Culpeper at the time, cayenne's healing powers are due to one chemical, **capsaicin**.

Cayenne became popular among early Americans after the Civil War, when a group of physicians known as Eclectics labeled the red pepper "capsicum" and used it topically to treat arthritis and sore muscles. They also found it to be useful in the treatment of colds, fever, diarrhea, nausea, toothache, delirium tremens, constipation, and cough.

Medicinal uses for cayenne have changed little since the days of the Eclectics. Cayenne facilitates digestion by stimulating the production of saliva and gastric juices, and it also stimulates the appetite; its antibacterial properties help relieve infectious diarrhea. Perhaps its most popular use is as a topical medicinal cream or ointment to relieve severe, chronic pain, especially that associated with shingles and diabetic foot pain. For these purposes, cayenne is available in two over-the-counter creams, Zostrix and Axsain. A topical capsaicin preparation is also effective in relieving the extreme pain associated with cluster headache. Preliminary study results also suggest cayenne may be useful in reducing cholesterol levels and treating heart disease. In a powder form, it can be sprinkled on bleeding wounds without causing pain or burning of the skin.

Cetyl Myristoleate (cerasomal-cis-9-cetylmyristoleate), or CMO, is a natural fatty acid found in certain animals. It is used as a supplement for treatment of arthritis and other autoimmune conditions. Proponents of CMO claim it can eliminate the cause of arthritis, stop the pain, and restore flexibility to the joints.

In 1971, researchers at the National Institutes of Health discovered CMO, then studied its effect in animals for approximately 10 years. One of the founders developed arthritis after leaving NIH and used CMO to treat himself. Results of his successful treatment were published in the *Journal of Pharmaceutical Sciences*.

CMO is an oily substance found in cows, beavers, mice, and whales. This oil is processed and converted into a powder for use in capsules. Reportedly, a twelve-day course of treatment with CMO produces dramatic relief from arthritic symptoms. It apparently achieves this by stopping the T-cells, which attack the body's joints, from their destructive behavior. The benefits of CMO are said to extend to both rheumatoid and osteoarthritis, lupus, multiple sclerosis, and other autoimmune disorders. Based on anecdotal evidence and limited studies by the NIH, no harmful side effects have been noted from use of CMO.

Chakras (SHAK-ras) (Sanskrit for ''wheels'') are the energy centers of the body, which absorb and release the life force, or **chi**. According to Eastern philosophies, there are seven chakras in the body: each one corresponds to an

THE BODY'S CHAKRAS

CHAKRA	COLOR	ASSOCIATED GLAND/ ORGAN
crown	violet	pineal
brow	indigo	pituitary
throat	blue	thyroid/parathyroid
heart	green	heart and thymus
navel/solar plexus	yellow	pancreas and adrenal
spleen	orange	spleen
root/sacral	red	sacrum, gonads, ovaries

endocrine gland and governs a specific area of the body. Each one also is associated with certain emotional issues and a particular color (see box).

Chamomile (or camomile) (KAM-e-mil) is not one herb but two that have long been used by Europeans and which are now popular in the United States. One is the German (or Hungarian) plant *(Matricaria chamomilla)*, and the other is the Roman (or English) plant *(Anthemis nobilis)*. Although these two plants are not related botanically, they have similar healing effects. Both plants grow in the United States, but the German variety is more common.

Chamomile tea, made from the dried yellow flowers of the plant, has traditionally been used to relieve stress and related conditions, such as nervous stomach, diarrhea, indigestion, and insomnia. It is also used to ease menstrual cramps and backache. Chamomile contains a chemical called bisabolol, an antispasm agent, which apparently is responsible for its soothing effect on digestive problems and menstrual cramps. In the fight against infection, chamomile has demonstrated the ability to kill the yeast that causes vaginal infections, *Candida albicans.* When applied as a poultice, it may relieve sore muscles and swelling, and a chamomile extract can ease skin irritation. Because chamomile belongs to the ragweed family, those who are sensitive to ragweed should avoid this herb.

Chaste Berries *(Vitex agnus castus)*, also known as chaste bush, chaste tree, and nunswort, were used in ancient times to suppress the libido of priestesses in the temples. It is still an important herb for women, though its primary use today is to relieve premenstrual syndrome and the symptoms of menopause.

Modern herbalists prescribe chaste berries to alleviate hot flashes, menstrual cramps, amenorrhea, and menopausal melancholia and to regulate menstrual cycles. Up to 90 percent of women who take a chaste berry remedy report relief of symptoms. After exhaustive studies, researchers at the University of Gottingen in Germany report that chaste berry regulates women's hormone balance, probably through its influence on the pituitary gland, which is responsible for the production and secretion of sex hormones. (They believe the herb's volatile oil is responsible for this action.) Some women who take chaste berry remedies for menstrual disorders who also have shingles or acne notice improvement in these disorders. It is uncertain why this benefit occurs.

Chelation Therapy (kee-LAY-shun) is a treatment method that removes toxic metals from the body. The word "chelation" evolved from the Greek word "chele," which means bind or claw. In chelation therapy, a nontoxic agent called EDTA (ethylene-diamine-tetra-acetate) is circulated through the body via an intravenous line. The EDTA bonds with, or chelates, with heavy metals and calcium in the body and eliminates them.

Chelation therapy is included in this volume because, although it is a medical procedure performed by allopathic and osteopathic physicians, it is a controversial therapy and is approved by the FDA solely for the treatment of heavy metal toxicity. However, some physicians use chelation therapy for patients with cardiovascular problems, including angina, hypertension, poor circulation, and breathing difficulties. For people with these conditions, EDTA bonds with calcium, which helps form the plaque that blocks arteries. Removal of excess calcium opens up the blood vessels and improves blood circulation. Chelation therapy also reportedly relieves symptoms of arthritis and may significantly reduce insulin requirements in people with diabetes. Some claims have been made that it is an effective cancer preventative and that it may slow the progress of Alzheimer's disease.

Chi (chee) in **Chinese medicine** (or *qi* in Japanese tradition) is the concept called the universal life force, universal energy, or vital energy. Chi is considered the basis of all life and ideally flows unhindered through all life forms. Chi is regulated and kept flowing by **yin and yang**, which, according to Chinese philosophy, governs all things in the universe.

Chi flows through invisible pathways called **meridians** and provides all the organs and systems of the body with energy. If chi is disrupted or hindered—as it can be by poor nutrition, excesses in lifestyle (e.g., lack of sleep, excessive alcohol or drug use, lack of exercise), environmental stressors, pollution, and emotional and physical trauma—the result is physical, emotional, mental, or spiritual dis-ease. Restoration and maintenance of the free flow of chi is the primary purpose of many forms of eastern holistic medicine and therapy.

The condition of the chi flow is instrumental in making a diagnosis in **traditional Chinese medicine**. Practitioners of Chinese medicine can feel the balance and flow of chi through people's meridians through a method of investigation called pulse diagnosis. To the trained diagnostician, the condition of the flow of chi also reveals any weaknesses in the body and can warn of potential problems. According to Chinese medicine, most of the diseases present in today's world are caused by a deficiency of chi. Practitioners of Chinese medicine emphasize the need to prevent chi deficiency by following good nutritional practices and adhering to a healthy lifestyle.

ALSO SEE acupressure; acupuncture; energy therapies

Chi Gong (chee gong) see qigong

Chi Nei Tsang (chee nay tong) means "transforming energy of the internal organs," and is also known as Internal Organs Integrated Massage. The focus of the therapy is on the navel area—which, according to Taoist philosophy, is where everything in the body originates—and the internal organs of the abdominal cavity.

In **Chinese medicine**, the **meridians**, the circulatory, nervous, and lymphatic systems, and the organs involved in digestion, elimination, and assimilation all cross paths in the abdominal cavity. This area is "command central" for the entire body: if it is out of balance, the effects are felt throughout the body. Chi nei tsang brings "command central" back into balance.

Unlike **shiatsu** and **acupuncture**, whose treatments indirectly stimulate the internal organs, chi nei tsang involves direct manipulation and **massage** of the organs. Practitioners of chi nei tsang use massage, **acupressure**, and breathing exercises to free up the flow of energy and eliminate toxins from the internal organs, bones, and tissues. This process can also balance the emotions, as the Taoists believe the internal organs also produce and store emotions.

To bring the organs back into balance and better functioning, practitioners of chi nei tsang use various hand and elbow techniques to pat, press, rub, rock, and otherwise manipulate the abdominal area. They also work the areas close to the spine to release tension, help correct postural problems, and stimulate the immune system.

Chinese Medicine

is a complex medical system that has been practiced for more than 2,000 years to treat hundreds of millions of people. Its beginnings have been traced to a book called *Nei Ching* (or *Nei Jing*), *The Yellow Emperor's Classic of Internal Medicine*, reportedly compiled by seven medical scholars before the time of Hippocrates.

Chinese medicine is nature-based, meaning that the same laws that govern nature and the universe are used to help practitioners understand the nature of the human body and its inner universe. Thus all people are viewed as part of and related to the greater environment and so are subject to the same laws, which center on balance and harmony.

At the core of Chinese medicine are the concepts of **chi** and **yin and yang**. Chi, which is the life-force energy that flows throughout the body, appears in two forms—yin and yang—complementary forms of chi. All people consist of a unique makeup of yin and yang. It is the premise of Chinese medicine that health prevails when yin-yang is balanced and flowing smoothly and that illness or disease occurs when there is blockage or interrupted flow. The goal of Chinese medicine, therefore, is to maintain or restore balance by affecting the flow of chi. This can be achieved using one or more practices, which include acupuncture/acupressure, nutrition, and Chinese herbal remedies.

Before Chinese medicine practitioners can prescribe any remedy, they need to determine their patients' yin-yang state. Examinations include pulse diagnosis—feeling the flow, or pulse, of chi through the major **meridians** at various sites on the wrist. Other diagnostic techniques include **tongue diagnosis**; observing body movement, posture, and general appearance; listening to the voice, breath, and abdominal sounds; noting breath and body odors and presence of perspiration; abdominal touch diagnosis; investigating sleep patterns; and urine analysis. Practitioners also determine their patients' mental and emotional states and evaluate their demeanors. All of the findings are used to create a complete picture of a patient's current state of balance and to determine a diagnosis and treatment plan. Treatment may include **acupressure**, **acupuncture**, **herbal medicine**, **nutritional therapies**, or **moxibustion**.

Several varieties of Chinese medicine are practiced in the United States; they include: **traditional Chinese medicine**, which is by far the most common; classical acupuncture, medical acupuncture, Japanese acupuncture, and auricular acupuncture. Many practitioners practice an eclectic mix of these traditions to suit the needs of individual patients. Chinese medicine has proved effective in treating a wide variety of diseases and symptoms, depending on the exact technique chosen. Generally, Chinese medicine is helpful in acute conditions such as flu, allergy, common cold, and headache, and in the treatment of dental, arthritic, menstrual, back, and chronic pains. It works best, however, as a preventive medicine.

ALSO SEE acupressure; cupping

Chiropractic (ki-ro-PRAK-tik) is the philosophy, science, and art of locating, analyzing, and correcting vertebral subluxations—misalignments or dislocations of a joint comprised of two vertebra. The key principle of chiropractic is that subluxations change the body's normal neurophysiological functioning. D.D. Palmer, a self-taught healer who developed chiropractic in 1895, believed that subluxations disrupt the flow of Innate Intelligence (Palmer's term for the life force), which flows within each of us through the nervous system and has the ability to restore health. Thus if one or more of the 24 vertebrae of the spinal column are injured, irritated, or misaligned, proper flow of the force is disturbed and pain, discomfort, or compromised functioning often occur at the body sites that correspond to the nerves that exit from the traumatized spinal region.

Chiropractic was born in Davenport, Iowa, when Palmer, a successful faith healer who had studied physiology and anatomy, was sought out by a man who had been deaf since he injured himself seventeen years earlier while working in a confined position. Palmer noticed a prominent vertebra in the man's upper spine, the site of the original injury. When Palmer repositioned the vertebra, the man's hearing returned. Palmer immediately began formulating his philosophy on what he called "chiropractic," which combines the Greek *cheir* ("hand") and *praxis* ("practice"). His original philosophy emphasized that any disease process is affected to some degree by the nervous system; thus any disease or ailment can be helped by chiropractic.

Chiropractors can be classified in several categories. "Straight" chiropractors limit their practice to the anatomy of the spine and vertebral subluxations. "Mixers," who make up the majority of chiropractors, integrate other modalities in their treatment practices. These commonly include nutritional supplementation, **Chinese medicine**, **naturopathy**, **massage** or **bodywork**, **homeopathy**, and other natural healing methods. Another variation, called "network chiropractic," utilizes a special system of twelve techniques as its treatment regimen.

Chiropractic is effective in treating neuromusculoskeletal problems, especially back and neck pain; headache and migraine; and conditions related to the knees, wrists, ankles, and other joints.

Choline (KO-leen) is a nutrient produced in the body and abundant in the phospholipid lecithin. Choline is touted for its ability to improve memory, treat Alzheimer's disease, reduce high blood pressure and cholesterol levels, and control mood swings. Because choline supplements break down in the intestines and cause fishy breath, people who want choline usually take it in the form of lecithin, which does not cause a fishy odor.

The body produces choline, an essential building block for acetylcholine, a chemical in the brain that transmits messages between nerve cells and is instrumental in developing cell membranes. Choline/lecithin is found naturally in oatmeal, soybeans, cauliflower, kale, cabbage, peanuts, eggs, seaweed, and chocolate. Choline/lecithin also is available in supplemental form, which many people are turning to because it reportedly can improve memory loss, especially in people with Alzheimer's disease. Some studies suggest that choline may protect the liver against alcohol damage.

Chondroitin Sulfate (kon-DROY-tin) is a substance found naturally in the body and which helps maintain the elasticity and integrity of many of the body's tissue systems, especially the connective tissue and blood vessel walls. It does this by attracting water to cartilage, which helps promote joint mobility and prevent premature breakdown of cartilage, and by inhibiting the activity of certain enzymes that destroy cartilage.

Recent research indicates that chondroitin sulfates may be effective in the treatment of arthritis. As people age, the water content of the cartilage decreases, causing problems in the joints. Malnutrition, arthritis, and trauma also can compromise the integrity of cartilage.

Supplementation with chondroitin sulfates to treat arthritis came to the fore with publication of the book *The Arthritis Cure*, by Jason Theodosakis, M.D., M.S., M.P.H., in the mid-1990s. Chondroitin sulfates are also used as a preventive agent for vascular disease.

The use of chondroitin sulfates alone can benefit those who suffer with osteoarthritis. However, some believe that the combination of chondroitin and **glucosamine sulfate**, another naturally occurring compound involved with maintaining healthy cartilage, works synergistically to stimulate cartilage production and helps control the destruction of cartilage.

Chodroitin sulfate is available in tablets and should be taken under the direction of a physician.

Chromium is an essential trace nutrient that plays an important role in the maintenance of blood sugar (glucose) levels and, in turn, increases energy levels. Although chromium is essential in the diet, the Food and Drug Administration (FDA) has not established a Recommended Daily Allowance (RDA). The best food sources of chromium include brewer's yeast, whole grains, beets and beet sugar, molasses, mushrooms, and mineral-rich hard water.

Chromium's part in regulating blood sugar levels makes it a critical nutrient to monitor in people with diabetes, because a deficiency in chromium can lead to elevated blood sugar levels, high blood cholesterol levels, and a buildup of plaque in the blood vessels. Researchers first discovered the link between chromium and glucose levels in 1955 when they gave brewer's yeast to glucose-intolerant rodents and the rats experienced normal glucose tolerance.

Therapeutically, supplemental chromium can improve glucose tolerance and increase sensitivity to insulin in people with Type II diabetes (noninsulin-dependent diabetes). Chromium is also reported to help cause weight loss, which may be associated with its ability to regulate blood sugar levels, which in turn reduces cravings for sugar. There are also reports that a form of chromium known as chromium picolinate may promote body fat loss and improve muscle development.

Another possible therapeutic use for chromium is in the prevention of atherosclerotic disease, or the accumulation of fatty deposits on the arteries. Chromium also may stimulate the body's production of **DHEA** (considered to be an important anti-aging hormone, help prevent some forms of dental cavities), and help protect against cancer of the esophagus.

Chua Ka (choo kah) is a form of deep tissue massage that is easy to self-administer. This ancient Mongolian body therapy, which means "to sculpture out," was practiced by Mongolian warriors before they went into battle to help purify their bodies of physical and emotional worry.

Chua ka is based on the idea that there are 27 "zones of karma" in the body, and each region stores a specific psychological fear. When people practice chua ka, they remove all accumulated fears and tensions from the zone in which it is stored, which leaves the body flexible and relaxed. Chua ka is used to release emotional stress and fear, relieve chronic tension and pain, reduce cellulite, increase awareness and flexibility, and facilitate healing after injury or illness.

ALSO SEE deep tissue massage

Coenzyme Q-10 (or Co-Q-10) is a natural substance in the body whose primary role is to assist enzymes (coenzymes are the "coworkers" of enzymes) in the metabolism and utilization of oxygen. It was discovered in 1957, and, based on recent research, it may warrant vitamin status, as it seems to be essential for effective oxygenation of the cells.

Coenzyme Q-10 is available as a supplement and is largely marketed as an **antioxidant**. Because of its ability to improve the utilization of oxygen, it is used by people with diabetes, poor circulation, coronary insufficiency, and multiple sclerosis. It also has been credited with alleviating and curing gum disease and other gum problems; boosting the immune system; and improving metabolism. Some individuals report that it helps increase aerobic endurance, improve strength, promote weight loss, and increase endurance.

Cognitive Therapy (CAHG-nuh-tiv) is an organized self-help technique in which people consciously restructure their negative emotions and feelings about themselves, their problems, and their life circumstances to allow them to get true, undistorted perspectives of particular situations. It was pioneered in the 1970s by Aaron Beck, M.D., and subsequently widely publicized and utilized by David D. Burns, M.D. Yet the premise on which it is based was recognized more than 2,000 years ago when the Greek philosopher Epictetus said, ''People are not disturbed by events themselves, but rather by the views they take of them.'' Today's cognitive therapists echo that view, claiming that most negative emotions are caused by distorted thinking.

Although some mental health problems are caused by chemical imbalances in the brain, and may best be treated with antidepressants, cognitive therapy is more effective than medication for people with mild to moderate depression and for those with anxiety, stress, feelings of guilt, and phobias.

Dr. Burns identified ten forms of distorted thinking which he claims cause people to struggle with negative emotions (see box). He also developed The Burns Anxiety Inventory, The Burns Depression Checklist, and other tools to help people identify their negative emotions. Once people identify their negative thinking patterns, they can take steps (and Dr. Burns has conveniently created seven such steps) to bring them back to clear, balanced thinking.

TEN FORMS OF DISTORTED THINKING

All-or-nothing thinking: You see things in extremes; something is either a complete success or a total failure; you either please everyone or are good for nothing. This is also known as "black-and-white" thinking.

Labeling: You put a name to how you feel about yourself. Instead of simply accepting that you made a mistake, you label yourself as an "idiot."

Overgeneralization: If you find yourself applying the words "forever," "always," or "never" to situations or events, you are probably overgeneralizing. "I'll never be any good" and "I'll be stuck in this line forever" are examples.

Mental filtering: This is the tendency to filter out all the positive factors and focus solely on the negative. Example: You've prepared a beautiful buffet, which everyone raves about, but one person remarks that the soup was too spicy. You decide you have failed.

Discounting the positive: If you think "I'm not good enough," "An idiot could have done what I did," or "What I did doesn't count," you're refusing to see the positive in what you do.

Jumping to conclusions: You make assumptions without any supporting evidence, or you predict the worst will happen in given situations.

Magnification: You greatly exaggerate any negative aspect of situations. For example, you get a flat tire and decide that your entire car is no longer any good.

Emotional reasoning: You mistakenly believe your emotions are reality. For example, you feel guilty about arriving late for a friend's dinner party, so you decide you are a bad person.

"Should" and "shouldn't" statements: You blame yourself by saying "I should have done better" or "I shouldn't have eaten that piece of cake." Words like "must," "have to," and "ought to" can be substituted as well.

Personalizing the blame: You take full responsibility for things over which you have little or no control. For example: You schedule a picnic, it rains, and you blame it on yourself.

Colloidal Silver (kol-OYD-al) is a liquid solution that contains submicroscopic particles of silver, held in suspension in pure water by the tiny electrical charge that is on each particle. It is a powerful antibiotic agent that has demonstrated its bacteria-killing effect against approximately 650 disease organisms.

The healing and medicinal benefits of silver have been known for centuries. Wealthy people in ancient civilizations stored their water in silver vessels to prevent the growth of bacteria, and this practice survived until colonial times in America, when settlers put silver dollars in milk containers to delay spoilage. In the late 1800s, Western researchers proved silver's bacteria-fighting properties, and a silver solution known as colloidal silver soon was introduced to the marketplace. (A "colloid" is a solution consisting of ultrafine particles suspended in liquid.) It remained a popular infection-fighting agent, but as the cost of silver rose, so did the motivation to find more cost-effective drugs to combat infection. As antibiotics were developed, use of colloidal silver diminished.

As problems with the effectiveness of antibiotics became apparent, the use of colloidal silver returned in the 1970s, and at a more economical cost. Investigations into the efficacy of colloidal silver show that it successfully treats many ailments and diseases, and without the adverse effects associated with other antibiotics. Conditions as diverse as pink eye, sinus infection, chronic fatigue syndrome, and cuticle infection can be treated successfully with colloidal silver. Some physicians include silver as a component in their cancer treatments.

Colon Hydrotherapy (KO-len hi-dro-THER-uh-pee) (also called colonic irrigation or colonic therapy) is the use of water as a method to flush out accumulated waste and toxins from the upper and lower portions of the large intestine, or colon. Because most people in industrialized societies consume a low-fiber, high-fat diet, putrefied feces often build up and become impacted in the colon. Over time this material may cause autointoxication, a condition in which the toxins in the decaying matter enter the bloodstream and poison the body. Many experts believe autointoxication causes various health problems, including colon cancer.

Colon hydrotherapy involves inserting a tube into the rectum and sending water (at body temperature) into the upper colon, where it flushes out bacteria, impacted feces, and other colonic debris. A second tube carries the water and waste from the body. During the process, which usually takes from 45 to 60 minutes, the colonic hydrotherapist massages the colon through the abdomen to help loosen impacted material. Some therapists also use **reflexology** or **acupressure** to assist the elimination process.

The procedure is considered dangerous by many practitioners because of the risk of introducing infectious agents, such as HIV, and because it removes good as well as bad bacteria. Colonic hydrotherapy should be performed only by professionally trained therapists who use meticulous sterilization methods. To address the issue of bacteria removal, many therapists use herbs and other substances to promote the growth of "good" bacteria in the colon. Supplements of **acidophilus** and bifidus—good bacteria that reside in the gut—are often recommended after treatment to restore a healthy colonic environment.

Unlike its predecessor, the enema, which has been documented as far back as 1500 B.C. in Egypt, modern colonic irrigation was introduced in the 1890s by Dr. Elmer Lee and written about in a book by Simon Baruch, M.D., called *The Principles and Practice of Hydrotherapy: A Guide to the Application of Water in Disease* (1898). After a brief stint as a therapy for people with arthritis, heart disease, depression, and other disorders, it lost favor in the 1940s when allopathic drug use surged. Today interest has returned and it is offered by naturopaths, colonic hydrotherapists, and other specially trained health-care professionals. ALSO SEE hydrotherapy

Color Therapy (also called color healing) is a form of energy therapy that involves the therapeutic use of different forms of color and light in order to promote and improve physical, spiritual, emotional, and mental well-being. Evidence of the use of color therapy has been found in ancient Egyptian manuscripts and in the works of Chinese and Indian mystics. It has long been a part of **Ayurvedic medicine**.

The eye filters normal daylight and produces the seven colors of the spectrum: red, yellow, orange, green, blue, indigo, and violet. Each color vibrates at its own frequency. The impact of these different colors on people has been recognized by health professionals for centuries (see box). The effects of color can be physical, psychological, and psychic. Some color therapists believe that as certain colors are absorbed through the skin, they can influence body chemistry, which can have both a physical and emotional impact. Another school of thought is that the colors themselves do not do the healing but that they provide the body with the stimulation to perform its own healing. In both cases, the premise is that color can increase the vibration rate of the body's cells, which naturally vibrate. Blue light reportedly lowers blood pressure, while red increases it. Specific colors in an environment also can have an effect. Hyperactive individuals who are put into rooms that have green or blue walls, for example, become noticeably calmer, while red and yellow have a calming effect on depressed patients.

Many color therapists work on a psychic level with a person's **aura**—an energy field that manifests as a haze or shimmering colored light around the body. The color of a person's aura depends on his or her physical, emotional, and spiritual state of being, thus it changes to reflect those conditions. Therapists also use color to influence the body's seven energy centers, or **chakras**. Each chakra corresponds to one of the colors of the light spectrum.

Scientific proof as to why color and light can heal is accumulating. Scientists have found that our cells are composed of contracted light, and we know that light responds to color, based on the vibrations emitted by any given color. Therapists choose colors that vibrate at the level required to balance the cells and promote healing at the cellular level.

ALSO SEE Ayurvedic medicine

COLOR	PROPERTIES AND EFFECTS
Red:	heating, stimulating; heals blood deficiency diseases; improves circulation; helps remove mucus and toxins
Orange:	stimulates the lungs; relieves convulsions, cramps, and gas
Yellow:	influences the higher mind and soul; helps loosen calcium and lime deposits; aids in food assimilation
Green:	vibration of balance and harmony; restores nervous system; stimulates the pituitary gland; represents the cleansing principle
Blue:	calm, peaceful vibrations; induces sleep and relaxation; can relieve inflammation, nervousness
Indigo:	treatment of some nervous and mental disorders; influences the area of the brain where the pineal gland is located
Violet:	highest vibrational rate; best for artistic and creative temperament

Comfrey (KUM-free) *(Symphytum officinale)* (common name, knitbone) is a very prolific plant whose primary healing powers are revealed in its common name: it has been used since ancient times as a poultice to heal fractures, sores, damaged tendons and ligaments, wounds, and skin ulcers. It apparently was given its alternative name because cloths soaked in comfrey paste harden like plaster casts when wrapped around broken bones. This was a common practice among soldiers in ancient times. Ancient Greek physicians also found that comfrey tea was effective in treating respiratory and gastrointestinal disorders.

The herb's ability to promote skin and bone healing is associated with a component called allantoin, which helps stimulate new cell growth and reduce inflammation. Traditional herbalists used comfrey as a tea or extract to purify the blood and to cure stomach ulcers. They also utilized its astringent properties to treat hemorrhaging, including bleeding hemorrhoids, and its high mucilage content to ease respiratory disorders and symptoms.

Some comfrey root and leaves (Russian comfrey *[S. uplandicum]* and prickly comfrey *[S. asperum]* in particular) contain significant amounts of pyrrolizidine alkaloids, which reportedly may cause liver damage if consumed in large amounts over an extended time. For this reason, some modern herbalists recommend comfrey be used only topically in ointments, creams, and poultices; other experts claim that small amounts of ingested comfrey are safe. There is some controversy over the results of a few studies that show that comfrey contains some cancer-causing substances. Comfrey also contains many cancer-fighting agents, so many modern herbalists still recommend comfrey for treatment of wounds as well as ulcers, ulcerative colitis, bronchitis, bleeding gums, digestive complaints, hoarseness, and internal hemorrhage. The Food and Drug Administration lists comfrey as being of "undefined safety."

Connective Tissue Massage is a **bodywork** therapy developed in Germany and based on the concept of trigger points (hypersensitive sites in the connective tissue and muscle). When a trigger point is stimulated, it affects the organs and tissues in another part of the body, and it also can refer pain to another site.

When performing connective tissue massage, the therapist hooks his or her fingers into the skin and superficial connective tissue and uses a pulling stroke to stretch the skin. This technique leaves a mark that resembles an abrasion, but this clears without a scar.

Connective tissue massage, which is also known as Bindegewebsmassage, was developed by Elizabeth Dicke, who, after learning she had a serious medical problem, experimented with different massage forms on herself. The result of her research was connective tissue massage. It is considered a physical therapy technique in Germany and a medical technique in many parts of Europe. In the United States, connective tissue massage is taught in many massage schools.

ALSO SEE massage

Contact Reflex Analysis (CRA) is a simple, natural method of muscle testing during which trained testers analyze the body's reflexes to accurately identify nutritional deficiencies. Nutritional deficiencies are associated with and contribute to various acute and chronic health problems. CRA is a tool that indicates the root cause of symptoms and health problems; it is not a diagnostic technique. CRA was researched and developed by Dr. R. Versendaal, C.D., along with a medical doctor, a clinical nutritionist, a dentist and a hematologist.

It is believed that when the body is out of harmony or balance, transmission of nerve energy to the reflexes throughout the body is interrupted. CRA practitioners (commonly called testers) can test a client's reflexes to determine if nerve energy is flowing freely. To test a reflex, a tester uses the client's arm muscle as an indicator. The client holds an arm out to the side, parallel with the floor. As the tester's finger touches or comes close to a healthy reflex somewhere on the body—one with free-flowing energy—the arm muscle remains strong when the tester applies downward pressure on it. If, however, the tester can easily push the arm down, this indicates a "break" in the flow of nerve energy. Once the deficiencies have been identified, professional CRA testers can recommend structural or nutritional support to regain balance.

Craniosacral Therapy (kray-nee-oh-SAK-ral) is a noninvasive, hands-on therapy that involves applying gentle pressure to the craniosacral system, which includes the skull, the face, and the spinal column down to the coccyx (tailbone). Within this system circulates the cerebrospinal fluid (CSF), which nourishes, protects, and bathes the brain, spinal cord, and nerve roots. Craniosacral therapy practitioners gently manipulate areas along the craniosacral system in order to release any restricted flow of the CSF and thus restore balance and well-being to the body and relieve pain, stress, and tension.

Craniosacral therapy evolved from osteopathy and originated in the 1920s and 1930s when William G. Sutherland, an osteopath, experimented with the application of pressure to various parts of the skull. To Dr. Sutherland, life is a series of movements, rhythms, and pulsations which he called "the breath of life." According to Sutherland, manipulation of the craniosacral system allows "the breath of life" to permeate the entire body. Dr. Sutherland published a book about his research of craniosacral osteopathy (called *The Cranial Bowl*), yet this therapy was largely ignored until the 1970s when John E. Upledger, D.O., explored craniosacral osteopathy and realized its potential in treating ailments as diverse as headaches and neuromuscular disorders, such as cerebral palsy.

Dr. Upledger explains that the movement of cerebrospinal fluid within the craniosacral system causes the bones of the skull to move as the pressure and volume of fluid change. If there are any blockages within the system, they can cause pain or dysfunction at various places in the body. Thus a craniosacral therapist first assesses the flow of CSF to determine where the flow is restricted and then manipulates sites along the system to free it.

Craniosacral therapy can be used to treat people who have migraine, chronic headache, high blood pressure, sinus problems, ringing of the ears, vision problems, insomnia, TMJ (Temporo-Mandibular Joint) syndrome, dizziness, Bell's palsy, nervous disorders, cerebral palsy and other types of paralysis, and back pain. It has been successful in helping children who have learning disabilities or who are hyperactive or dyslexic.

Craniosacral therapy is typically practiced by health-care professionals who are also osteopaths, medical doctors, chiropractors, physical and occupational therapists, dentists, and massage therapists. Both adults and children can benefit from craniosacral therapy; work on infants needs to be done by a professional who is specially trained in working with them.

ALSO SEE osteopathy

Crystal and Gem Healing (also called crystal therapy or gem therapy) involves the use of gemstones, quartz crystals, and other types of natural crystals and stones for therapeutic purposes. The basis for their use in healing is the belief that the Earth's magnetic field is composed of the vibrational energy of crystals and gemstones, as is the magnetic field of the human aura. At the same time, about one-third of the Earth is composed of crystal (in the form of silica and water). Thus humans, the Earth, and the crystals and gems in the Earth have similar energy and vibrational fields, which can be balanced for healing.

The healing powers of stones have been appreciated since primitive times and by many cultures. In the United States, Native Americans have a long history of using crystals for healing, but popular general interest didn't emerge until the 1980s. Stones and crystals are either worn on the body or placed in specific places in a person's environment to facilitate energy flow, restore energy balance, or unblock "stuck" energy. Gems and crystals are positioned over a **meridian** or on or near a **chakra** point. This placement allows the electromagnetic energy emitted by the stones to have the maximum impact on the flow of energy at those points of the body. Crystals can be used alone or in conjunction with chakra balancing and **color therapy**.

According to healers who use gems and crystals, the stones absorb energy from anyone who touches them, which includes negative energy, such as pain and disease, as well as positive. A stone that has not been "cleared"— cleansed of any energy it may have picked up from anyone who has handled it—can transmit that energy to the next person who holds the stone. Stones can be cleared in various ways, including soaking them in salt water, placing them under a pyramid, and burying them in the ground. Stones must be fully cleared in order for them to emit their most positive vibrations and heal.

The act of placing crystals and gemstones on or around a person (called a receiver) is called a "laying on of stones." When cleared stones are used, this therapy can cleanse the body of negative energy, clear and balance the chakras, replenish low levels of positive energy, and unblock "stuck" energy. Laying on of stones can also cause the receiver's vibrations to align with those of the Earth, placing the receiver in harmony with the Universe, freeing his or her life force energy, and transforming negative energy into health.

Crystal and gemstone therapy can accelerate the healing of wounds and injuries, reduce stress and symptoms associated with stress-related disorders, alleviate chronic or fatal conditions, and relieve pain.

Cupping is a Chinese therapeutic technique in which a small cuplike object is heated inside by a flame and then quickly placed on the skin. This action creates a vacuum, and the heated vacuum increases blood circulation and mobility in the area being treated. The cups are usually left in place for 10 to 15 minutes and then removed. Cupping is sometimes used along with **acupuncture** and **moxibustion**.

In ancient China, the cupping method was used to dispel pus and was called the "horn method" because animal horns were used. Today, both glass and bamboo jars are common. Cupping is effective in treating back pain, rheumatism, arthritis, and stiff muscles and joints.

ALSO SEE Chinese medicine

Cymatic Therapy (si-MAY-tik) is a form of **sound therapy** in which handheld devices, pads, or plates which emit high-frequency sounds are applied to specific parts of the body. It is believed that the vibrations and stimulation transmitted by the instruments possess healing effects.

Cymatic therapy was developed by Dr. Peter Manners in the 1960s. It is used in orthopedic units to facilitate treatment of bone fractures. It is also used to treat arthritis, gout, lower back pain, rheumatism, sciatica, slipped disc, sports injuries, stress-related muscle tension, and aid postsurgical

Dance Therapy (also called dance movement therapy) is a nonverbal form of communication that allows individuals to increase awareness of their feelings and learn to express them in a physical way. It is used primarily for people who have emotional or psychological problems, communication difficulties, or learning disabilities, or who are mentally ill.

Use of dance to help people with emotional problems was pioneered by dance and movement specialists Rudolph von Laban and Marian Chase in the 1940s. Laban, a pioneer physiotherapist and choreographer, believed that dance can affect parts of the mind that verbal communication cannot. He developed Laban-notation, a system of choreographic notation that dance therapists use to analyze the movements of their clients.

Participants in dance therapy do not need to know how to dance. Therapists encourage individuals to freely express themselves with their own movements and, if they wish or are able, to voice any emotions they may feel while dancing.

Dance therapy is often used with children and adolescents, although adults also participate. Conditions that respond to dance therapy include depression, schizophrenia, eating disorders, sleep disorders, headache and migraine.

Dandelion *(Taraxacum officinale)* is a low-growing, flowering perennial plant often regarded as a weed. This prolific plant has been used for healing for more than 1,000 years throughout India, the Middle East, and Europe. Its diuretic properties (ability to promote urination) were discovered by Arab physicians in the tenth century. Since ancient times, the Chinese have used dandelion to treat colds, ulcers, bronchitis, pneumonia, hepatitis, obesity, dental problems, and internal injuries. When the colonists came to North America, they brought dandelions with them and introduced the herb to the Native Americans, who used it as a tonic.

Today, dandelion is used in the United States primarily as a diuretic to treat premenstrual syndrome, menstrual symptoms, swollen feet, high blood pressure, and congestive heart failure. It is also used for weight loss, although it is not recommended as a dietary aid because the weight lost is due to water loss and therefore usually returns.

Deep Tissue Massage is a general term for a type of **bodywork** in which the deep layers of muscle and connective tissue are manipulated down to the bone. Several massage techniques fall into this broad category, including

rolfing, deep tissue sculpting, **Hellerwork**, and **chua ka**, among others.

All forms of deep tissue massage share several characteristics. Unlike full-body massage techniques, deep tissue massage usually focuses on releasing tension in a specific area of the body. In order to be effective, practitioners need to relax each layer of muscle as they work down to the bone. This usually involves use of the elbows and thumbs as well as the fingers. They also often direct their movements across the grain of the muscles (referred to as "cross-fiber massage"). All of these techniques allow deep tissue massage to relieve chronic muscular pain, reduce pain associated with arthritis and tendonitis, and help remove toxins and other waste materials from the muscles and surrounding tissues.

DHEA (dehydroepiadrosterone) is a hormone produced by the adrenal gland and is the most abundant hormone in the human bloodstream. It is used by the body to make dozens of other hormones, including the sex hormones. In addition to its role in hormone production, it plays a significant part in the immune system as an **antioxidant**, reduces the severity of allergic reactions, facilitates tissue repair, and is an anticancer agent.

DHEA is called a "superhormone" and is touted as an anti-aging and anti-obesity wonder by advertisers. It is credited with having a beneficial effect on people with diabetes, multiple sclerosis, and lupus. Some physicians say it protects the brain cells from Alzheimer's disease and other brain dysfunction.

DHEA has been the subject of more than 10,000 papers, two international conferences, and countless studies in both animals and humans, and many of the claims made appear to be true, at least to some extent. At the University of Arizona in Tucson, Ronald Watson, a research professor at the university's college of medicine, says his study results show "DHEA appears to lower heart disease risks and boost immune function in older humans." Julian Whitaker,

M.D., author of *Reversing Diabetes* and editor of *Health and Healing* newsletter, says "adequate DHEA ... can slow the aging process, prevent, improve, and even often reverse conditions such as cancer, heart disease, memory loss, obesity and osteoporosis ... DHEA is the closest we can get to the fountain of youth." Elizabeth Barret-Conner, M.D., of the University of California School of Medicine, reports that "DHEA seems to protect people against early death from any cause."

Caveats are also in order. Experts warn that DHEA is a hormone and should be treated as a potent medication. Much is still not known about it, although one serious adverse effect has been noted. People with a personal or family history of any type of tumor development that responds to hormones, such as prostate or breast cancer, should not take DHEA. Less critical side effects include fatigue, acne, irritability, insomnia, oily skin, and facial hair growth in some women.

DHEA is available over the counter and is marketed as a synthetic product or as containing animal extracts. At this time, there are no natural alternatives. Although a compound called diosgenin, found in wild yams, is claimed to be a precursor (a substance from which another substance is formed) to DHEA, it doesn't convert to DHEA in the body.

DMSO (dimethyl sulfoxide) is a byproduct of wood produced during papermaking that is available in several grades: commercial, pharmaceutical, and veterinarian. The pharmaceutical grade, suitable for human use, has dozens of therapeutic purposes.

DMSO, a slightly oily liquid that has a mild garlic odor and looks like mineral oil, was first synthesized in 1866 by a Russian scientist named Alexander Saytzeff. Though the commercial grade is commonly used as antifreeze and as a degreaser and paint thinner, the pharmaceutical solution, safe for human use, is reportedly effective in treating conditions as diverse as diabetes, Down's syndrome, and herpes. A popular use for DMSO is in the treatment of arthritis and rheumatism. Topical use of DMSO may relieve pain, reduce swelling and stiffness, and eliminate redness from affected joints.

DMSO reportedly can kill the bacteria that causes Lyme disease and the yeast that causes candidiasis. Injections of DMSO may eliminate sciatica and lower back pain, and intravenous DMSO along with chemotherapy can shrink tumors. Topical application of DMSO is credited with eliminating headache pain, healing varicose ulcers, and relieving the pain associated with sprains, pulled muscles, dislocated joints, burns, shingles, bunions, corns and calluses, and plantar warts. A dilution of DMSO ingested by children with Down's syndrome reportedly restores brain function to normal. For people with cataracts, DMSO may dissolve the growths without the need for surgery. There are also reports that DMSO is effective in the treatment of chronic fatigue syndrome, glaucoma, and diabetes.

DMSO is usually used and prescribed by naturopaths and osteopaths, and less often by medical doctors.

Do-In (du-in) is a form of self-acupressure and self-massage that involves breathing, stretching, and massage of **acupressure** points. It originated more than 5,000 years ago when Chinese Taoist monks noted that people in pain would hold or touch their injured or painful body part to heal themselves. The monks then developed a system called Tao-Yinn: Tao means "the way" and Yinn, "a gentle approach." Do-in was introduced to the United States by **macrobiotics** pioneer Michio Kushi, where it is used to maintain overall health and well-being and treat physical ailments such as neck and back pain, muscle tension, and arthritis.
ALSO SEE massage

Dowsing is used by some natural therapists for medical and healing purposes, to help them make assessments of their clients' health state. A dowser holds a pendulum over the body's **chakras**, or energy centers, to detect strengths and weaknesses in the body's energy flow. A pendulum also is used to obtain yes and no answers to specific questions about the client's health: a clockwise rotation indicates "yes" and a counterclockwise rotation indicates "no" to posed questions. It is important that the dowser's mind remain open and free of "intruding" thoughts, as strong opinions can unconsciously affect the pendulum's motion and result in false readings.

Dowsing for medical reasons was introduced in Western culture by a Frenchman named Abbe Mermet in the 1920s. Mermet believed that all things, including people, emit radiation. To identify this energy, Mermet developed radiesthesia, which means "sensitivity to radiations." Radiesthesia is performed using a pendulum as explained above.

Dream Therapy (also termed dream work) involves the interpretation of dreams and active participation in the dreaming process as a way to gain greater insight into behavior, emotions, physical ailments, and creative potential. The power of dreams and their meanings have fascinated people for thousands of years. The ancient Greeks believed dreams have the power to heal and built dream temples to cure the sick. Talented people from many different disciplines say they owe their creations to dreams, including Mozart, Billy Joel, Jack Nicklaus, Beethoven, Elias Howe (inventor of the sewing machine), Robert Louis Stevenson, and William Styron.

Although dreams have long captured our attention, scientific investigation of the dreaming process began relatively recently, in 1952, with the work of Nathaniel Kleitman, Ph.D., a physiology professor at the University of Chicago, and William Dement, M.D., Ph.D., who pioneered work with rapid eye movement (REM) sleep and its identification as "dream sleep." We know that dreams originate in the primitive part of the brain called the pons, and that dream activity is manifested as extremely fast, erratic nerve impulses that shoot from the pons to the part of the brain that produces emotion and reason. We still don't know, however, why we dream.

Most people interpret their own dreams, while some seek help from psychotherapists or dream analysts. Dream interpretation is usually sought to help people resolve emotional or spiritual matters. To solve a physical or emotional problem, you can actively participate in the dreaming process. This approach, called lucid dreaming, takes practice. It involves taking your conscious mind into the dream state. Once in that state, there is a moment when you are aware you are dreaming. At that time, you can influence your dream by saying a prearranged statement, such as ''help me heal my back pain.''

Many experts liken lucid dreaming to creative visualization, only better, because in lucid dreaming things seem more real. Lucid dreaming allows you to practice or test ideas or situations in a safe setting and then remember the results upon waking. Some athletes, for example, test new moves or strategies in their dreams before trying them in ''real'' life. Writers, inventors, business people, musicians, teachers—most people, with practice, can use lucid dreaming to tap into their creative energy, solve problems, dispel phobias, or work on any aspect of self-improvement.

Ear Coning (or ear candling) is an ancient technique using hollow candles to remove wax and other debris from the ears. It is also believed to be effective in removing bacteria, yeasts, fungi, candida, and remnants of past infections. It is more comfortable and less expensive than ear cleaning methods that force water into the ear canal, and can be done on people of all ages, including infants.

Ear coning probably originated with the Egyptians, who used it for spiritual as well as physical cleansing. They used hollow reeds to open and clear the spirit centers and refresh the **aura**s. Today, coning or candling is done with hollow candles that resemble large straws and are usually made of muslin coated with purified paraffin or beeswax. Some candles contain herbs or oils.

During a basic candling procedure, the face and hair are covered and protected before a candle is placed snugly into the ear. The candle must be snug to allow proper air draw to occur. As the candle burns, a vacuum is caused by the warmed air from the flame and the cooler air moving through the hollow candle. This suction action draws wax and other debris from the ear into the bottom of the candle.

In addition to removing wax buildup, ear candling is used as a last resort in children with chronic ear infections to avoid ear tubal placement. Candling also is effective in the treatment of earache, fluid in the ear, sinus congestion, headache, and dizziness, and it can remove impurities in the sinus and lymph systems. Some people report that it helps prevent colds by helping to clear toxins from the body.

Echinacea (ek-ih-NAY-see-uh) (*Echinacea angustifolia, E. purpurea, E. pallida*, and other species), also known as the purple coneflower or snakeroot, is a plant that is native to the central United States. It shares family affiliation with the daisy, marigold, and **dandelion**. Nine species grow in the United States, although the most commonly used species is *E. purpurea*. Much beloved by the Native Americans of the Great Plains, it was used to treat wounds, snakebites, toothaches, and sore throat. The early pioneers quickly noticed this herb's value in fighting infection, and by the late nineteenth century, a pharmaceutical company—Lloyd Brothers of Cincinnati—had added echinacea products to its line. The herb remained popular as an infection fighter until the 1930s, when the introduction of antibiotics caused the herb to lose favor in the United States. In Europe, however, researchers continued to both use and study it.

Today, echinacea has regained recognition and use in the United States in several areas. As a fighter of infection and inflammation, it is used to treat boils, eczema, poison oak and poison ivy, psoriasis, and other skin eruptions, as well as bladder infections, tonsillitis, and candida, a common chronic fungal infection. Echinacea also boosts the immune system, as it prevents the formation of hyaluronidase, an enzyme that destroys the body's natural defenses against viruses, fungi, and bacteria. Some people who undergo chemotherapy use echinacea to help restore normal immune functioning. Echinacea also can help reduce symptoms of cold or flu.

Egoscue Method (EE-go-sku) is a type of movement therapy based on the idea that in many people pain, lack of energy, stiffness, poor balance, and other physical dysfunction are caused by lack of motion or inadequate motion. According to its creator, Peter Egoscue, poor and lost physical functioning can be restored when the right kind and amount of movement are performed. Says Egoscue: We "are not moving enough to keep [our] body and overall health from deteriorating."

The Egoscue Method includes specific movements and exercises designed to systematically reintroduce highly focused, proper physical demands to dysfunctional muscle groups. Before exercise plans can be developed for people, their posture and movement need to be assessed. Egoscue has identified four basic body conditions, and every person fits into one of them. They are: (1) Hips tilted forward, which forces the head forward and the feet to turn outward; (2) hips tilted left to right with one side higher than the other and rotated, causing one hip to be forward, one shoulder to be higher than the other, and the head to hang forward; (3) head jutted forward, rounded and drooping shoulders, hips tilted under, flattened X-curve in the lower back, and the backs of the hands facing forward; and

(4) ideal body, with proper alignment from the head to the ankles, all joints level.

Each of the conditions has a specific sequence of exercises to be followed. The purpose of each exercise is to move the client from condition 1, 2, or 3 to body condition 4. The Egoscue Method can be effective in treating back and neck pain, musculoskeletal disorders, arthritis, and postural problems. It can help strengthen, stretch, and relax the body, increase flexibility, and relieve stress and tension.

Elderberry *(Sambucus canadensis)*, also known as American elder, is a small tree that is native to North America. There is also a European elder *(Sambucus nigra)* that grows in Europe, Asia, and North Africa, and which has been naturalized in the United States.

The elderberry tree has earned the distinction of the name "the medicine chest of the common people" because all of its parts have been used in traditional folk medicine for centuries. The berries contain more vitamin C than any other herb except rosehips and black currant, and also contain vitamins A and B as well as tannins, **carotenoids**, **amino acids**, and **flavonoids**.

The ancient Egyptians used the flowers to heal burns and improve the complexion. British citizens in the seventeenth century used elderberry wine to cure the common cold and prolong life. Many cultures have used the juice from the berries to cure colds, sore throat, and flu and to relieve bronchitis and asthma. Infusions of the fruit are credited with alleviating nervous disorders, back pain, and inflammation of the bladder and urinary tract.

Elderberry leaves contain many beneficial agents that may explain the herb's healing properties; these include the flavonoids rutin and quercetin; alkaloids; vitamin C; free fatty acids; potassium nitrate, and other substances. The flowers have a mild astringent property and are effective when used in skin washes to relieve eczema, acne, and psoriasis, or as an eye wash.

Electroacupuncture is a new form of **acupuncture** in which the acupuncture needles are stimulated with a weak electrical current. One popular form of this procedure is called "Ryodoraku," a method that originated in Japan but which has been adopted by many Western acupuncturists as an alternative approach to conventional "hands-on" treatments. Ryodoraku involves transmitting a weak electrical current through a clip that is attached to acupuncture needles. Proponents claim that the electrical stimulation promotes circulation and releases blocked energy. Electroacupuncture is believed to be effective in the treatment of pain.

Electrocrystal Therapy is a form of energy therapy that restructures energy flow to return it to a balanced state so the body can heal itself. It was developed in the 1970s by a British researcher, Harry Oldfield, who was also instrumental in the clinical use of **Kirlian photography**.

Electrocrystal treatment involves placing crystals in sealed glass tubes, which are filled with a brine solution. The tubes are placed on the relevant **chakras** and affected **meridians** of the patient, and an electric current is passed through the tubes. Healing is said to occur as the vibrations from the energized crystals pass through the body. Treatment is painless and completely safe. Electrocrystal therapy reportedly can relieve a wide variety of symptoms and improve many diseases, from headache to multiple sclerosis. ALSO SEE crystal and gem healing

Elimination Diet is the systematic exclusion of specific foods from the diet as a way to identify which ones are triggering adverse reactions. Food intolerances or sensitivities are believed to affect at least 10 percent of people, although some experts place that figure much higher. Symptoms of food intolerance can include headache, indigestion, mouth sores, diarrhea, constipation, irritable bowel, muscle and/or joint pain, bloating, flatulence, mental fogginess, and fatigue.

Food intolerance was first documented in 1888, when Dr. S.J. Gee published his findings about people who had adverse reactions to gluten (e.g., wheat, barley, oats, rye) and foods that contain these ingredients. This information was basically ignored until after World War II when doctors noted that the lack of wheat products in the Dutch diet "cured" many people of digestive problems, all of which returned when wheat was reintroduced.

Other foods that often trigger intolerance reactions are milk and dairy products, corn, and oranges; others include soy, MSG and other food additives, caffeine, high-fat foods, white potatoes, and peppers.

Not all elimination diets are created equal. The most vigorous form starts with a water-only fast and then allows one new food to be introduced into the diet each week. Other forms involve two food lists: foods allowed and those not allowed (those suspected of being part or all of the problem). After eating "allowed" foods for a period of time, "forbidden" foods are reintroduced one at a time, and reactions noted. Elimination diets can be time-consuming, but the information gathered from them may eliminate a lifetime of symptoms.

Energy Therapies are therapeutic methods based on the philosophy that all people consist of a subtle energy system that intimately connects their physical, emotional, mental, and spiritual states of being and that all these factors must be addressed when diagnosing and treating patients. The idea that people are energy has its roots in many Eastern philosophies and medical systems as well as religions and is now being supported by recent research into quantum physics.

The foundation of energy therapies is the idea that energy flows within the body through pathways called **meridians** and through energy centers called **chakras**. To maintain good health and well-being, it is necessary for energy to flow freely through the meridians and chakras. Physical, emotional, and mental illness and disease occur when the

energy flow is blocked or hindered. Some of the energy therapies used to maintain or restore energy flow include **acupuncture, applied kinesiology, biodynamic massage, qigong, color therapy, craniosacral therapy, crystal and gem healing, homeopathy, light therapy, polarity therapy,** spiritual/psychic healing, **shiatsu, sound therapy,** and **zero balancing**.
ALSO SEE Kirlian photography

Ephedra (ih-FED-ruh) is a term often used to describe any of several species of an herb that is a powerful bronchial decongestant. *Ephedra sinica*, a Chinese herb also known as *ma huang* or Chinese ephedra, and an American variety known as Mormon tea or desert tea *(Ephedra vulgaris)* are two of the more common species of this herb, which is considered by herb experts to be the world's oldest medicine. Chinese physicians are believed to have been prescribing ephedra tea to treat respiratory ailments since approximately 3000 B.C. Chinese ephedra is grown in the Inner Mongolia region of China. The American variety, which was discovered by early American pioneers and Mormon settlers, can be found in dry regions of North America.

Chinese ephedra contains a large amount of two alkaloids known as ephedrine and pseudoephedrine, which makes ephedra useful in the treatment of respiratory conditions such as asthma, bronchitis, allergies, common cold, and cough, and associated symptoms, such as watery eyes, stuffy nose, headache, and fever. Pseudoephedrine is a standard ingredient in conventional decongestants. American ephedra, however, usually does not contain these compounds, and when it does it's at much lower levels.

In Asia, Chinese ephedra is also commonly used as a coffeelike stimulant. In people who are seriously obese, Chinese ephedra can stimulate an increase in metabolic rate, causing some weight loss. This effect does not occur in individuals who are not greatly overweight. **Caution:** Because it may cause serious adverse effects, including convulsions, coma, and death, ephedra should only be taken under a physician's supervision.

Esalen Massage is a gentle form of bodywork that is more sensual than clinical in nature than are other forms of massage. It has been described as a synthesis of the best techniques from various styles of Eastern and Western massage. It was developed during the 1960s at the Esalen Institute in Big Sur, California, a center where self-growth and human potential are emphasized and promoted, and it has practitioners throughout the United States.

Soft, light, flowing strokes that cover the entire body are characteristic of Esalen massage. Practitioners of Esalen massage focus on providing a nurturing, relaxed, caring environment during their sessions. Benefits of Esalen massage may include reduced pain and stress, improved sleep, accelerated healing, and better digestion.
ALSO SEE massage

Essential Fatty Acids are fats the body needs to function optimally, but because it cannot manufacture them itself, they must be obtained through diet. Their primary role in the body is to strengthen cell membranes and facilitate the growth of nerves and muscles. Therapeutically, they have anti-inflammatory properties and may help to prevent heart disease. There is some evidence that they may also help to prevent cancer.

The essential fatty acids that have specific healing abilities include the omega-3s, such as eicosapentaenoic acid (EPA) and docosahexaenoic acid (DHA), and the omega-6s, including linoleic acid and gamma linolenic acid (GLA). The omega-3s are found in fish oils, particularly cold-water fish, and in hemp seed oil. Of the omega-6s, GLA is widely used as a supplement. Common sources include plant oils, such as **evening primrose**, borage, flax seed, rape seed, hemp seed, and black currant. Both omega-3 and omega-6 fatty acids have similar healing properties, which include the ability to reduce inflammation, lower blood fat and cholesterol levels, and thin the blood. These actions make them potentially beneficial in the treatment of arthritis, asthma, allergies, skin conditions, premenstrual syndrome, hypertension, and heart conditions.

Essential fatty acids do their good work by acting on prostaglandins, fatty acids produced by the body. Prostaglandins regulate various bodily processes, including blood pressure, cholesterol and triglyceride levels, and fluid balance. Sufficient levels of essential fatty acids help ensure the formation of the ''good'' prostaglandins as well as helping to lower total cholesterol levels.

Essential Oils are extremely concentrated substances, extracted from plants, that contain nearly all of a plant's nutrients, **amino acid** precursors, **minerals**, enzymes, **vitamins**, hormones, and other substances. These oils are the agents used in **aromatherapy** for both healing and cosmetic purposes. The use of essential oils dates back to approximately 3000 B.C.

Because essential oils are so concentrated, most of them are at least 50 times more powerful than the plants from which they are taken. Most essential oils contain dozens and sometimes hundreds of different chemicals, which makes it difficult to uncover all of their properties.

Essential oils enter the body either through inhalation or absorption through the skin. Inhalation can include breathing in the vapors from a bottle of oils or from a cloth or tissue treated with them; adding the oils to a vaporizer or bowl of hot water and breathing in the fragrance; or misting a room, office, or other indoor area with a mixture of oils and water. For skin absorption, the oils can be mixed with a carrier oil and applied directly to the skin in a compress or as a massage oil, or the oils can be added to bathwater and enter the skin while recipients soak in the tub.

Scientists believe that when essential oils are inhaled, the olfactory nerve transports the aroma to areas in the brain that control emotions and hormonal response. The chemicals in the oils may then cause a change in how individuals respond to or perceive symptoms. When they enter through the skin, the oils are absorbed into the tissues and the lymphatic system in about 20 minutes. The oils then travel in the body's fluids and carry their nutrients directly into the body's cells.

Depending on the essential oil used, they may have antibacterial, antifungal, antiviral, antiseptic, anti-inflammatory, and immune-boosting abilities. Essential oils are used to treat many conditions; for example, headache, muscle tension, stress, depression, anxiety, insomnia, premenstrual syndrome, menstrual cramps, asthma, common cold, flu, ulcers, sinusitis, bacterial infections, fatigue, hypertension, and muscle pain. They are also used to revitalize, nourish, and soften the skin.

Eucalyptus (yoo-kuh-LIP-tus) *(Eucalyptus globulus)* is an aromatic plant that yields a therapeutic oil commonly used for respiratory conditions. It has been used for millennia by the Australian aborigines for its antiseptic and healing properties. The active ingredient believed responsible for the plant's healing abilities is called eucalyptol.

Eucalyptus oil is a decongestant and is used to strengthen the respiratory system and build energy. Herbalists and aromatherapists use it to treat sinusitis, colds, flu, asthma, bronchitis, and allergies. Eucalyptus tea or cough drops are popular for relieving sore throat and cough.

Euphrasia (yoo-FRAY-she-uh) *(Euphrasia officinalis)* is a popular herbal remedy also known as **eyebright**. In **homeopathy**, it is used to treat various symptoms, including fever with chills; headache with eye complaints; excessive, watery discharge from the eyes, and a runny nose; burning pressure in the eyes accompanied by itching; and cough during the day, often accompanied by hoarseness in the morning. Generally, symptoms are worse in the daytime and are better when lying down. Because euphrasia is primarily a first aid remedy, no extensive psychological profile has been established for its homeopathic use.

Evening Primrose *(Oenothera biennis)*, a yellow-flowering plant in the willow family, native to North America, which some consider to be a weed, is an herb. It has a long history of use in America as both the Native Americans and early settlers used this plant to treat a wide range of conditions such as pain, asthma, and stomach disorders. Recent interest in this herb, however, is associated with the fact that the seeds contain a high percentage of an agent known as *cis*-gamma-linolenic acid (GLA), or omega-6 fatty acids, a key ingredient in the body's ability to produce prostaglandin E1 (a hormone essential for many bodily functions).

Ingestion of GLA in the form of evening primrose oil has been credited with lowering high blood pressure and high blood cholesterol levels, relieving premenstrual pain, reducing hangover symptoms, relieving rheumatoid arthritis, slowing the progression of multiple sclerosis, alleviating anxiety, and helping people lose weight without dieting. Most evening primrose oil is produced in Great Britain and is still considered to be "experimental" in the United States, although it is available.

Eyebright *(Euphrasia officinalis)* is a small annual plant native to Europe and England that is commonly used to treat eye ailments. It derives its name from the "bloodshot" look associated with the spots and lines on its flowers.

Since the Middle Ages, eyebright has been used to treat inflammation, especially of the eye and sinuses. Conditions relieved with eyebright include sinus congestion, eyestrain, conjunctivitis, eye inflammation, and itchy eyes due to colds or allergies. It also may help maintain good vision and overall eye health.

Many different compounds have been identified in the eyebright plant, but as yet none have been definitively linked with any of its healing effects. It does contain a tannin compound that has some anti-inflammatory properties. Eyebright is available in health and natural food

stores and is often found in combination with **goldenseal**, **echinacea**, or fennel seeds.
ALSO SEE bilberry

Eye-Robics is a vision-training technique that helps people improve their vision problems without the need for glasses, contact lenses, or invasive procedures. This self-help program was developed by Jerriann J. Taber, Ph.D., who learned and expounded upon the research and techniques of William H. Bates, M.D., and Margaret Darst Corbett.

The fundamental concept behind Eye-Robics is the belief that mental and emotional stress causes problem eyesight and that proper relaxation of the mind and body can restore imperfect sight and eliminate light sensitivity, which is the first sign of tension in the eyes and mind. In particular, the Eye-Robics program focuses on relaxation of the six intrinsic eye muscles, which allows the lens to reshape itself and in turn enables normal vision to return.

All vision problems are thought to be related to the nerves, and the Eye-Robics program addresses the cause—not the symptoms—of vision difficulties. The exercises are designed to allow participants to accept and receive light safely, keep their eyes relaxed, encourage imagining, and promote the integration of the left and right sides of the brain. When the eyes are relaxed, circulation improves and the eyes have the opportunity to correct their defects and build up resistance against future problems.

Eye-Robics can be practiced as a preventive approach for people with normal vision who want to guard against eyestrain and tension and for those who are entering a field that involves eyestrain. The program teaches how to read without strain and to handle stress visually by doing eye exercises which then allow the eyes to improve while they are working. The program includes visualization techniques that stimulate use of the mind's eye and enhance visual memory and imagination. As a healing therapy, Eye-Robics can improve near- and farsightedness, astigmatism, lazy eye, lack of depth perception, eyestrain, and excessively dry eyes. It may help people with cataracts, glaucoma, and macular degeneration.

ALSO SEE Bates Method of Vision Training

Fasting (medicinal) is a voluntary, controlled abstinence from solid foods for a specified amount of time. No fast should exclude liquids. Fasting is recommended by many health experts because it allows the body to cleanse itself of toxins that have accumulated from poor eating habits, polluted environment, and suppressed or repressed emotions; accelerates the healing process and stimulates the immune system; gives the digestive system an opportunity to rest; and desensitizes the body to food allergens. Fasting as a way to restrict calorie intake has been scientifically proven to extend life expectancy in animals and is believed to have the same effect in humans.

A study conducted in 1993 showed that fasting increases the body's levels of the "good" cholesterol, high-density lipoproteins (HDL). Gentle, healing activities such as **meditation**, **breathing therapies**, and **hydrotherapy** are sometimes done during a fast to enhance its benefits. Fasting is also credited with providing spiritual cleansing. Said Gandhi: "Fasting brings spiritual rebirth." Naturopaths usually recommend doing one 24- to 48-hour fast per month as a cleansing and preventive care measure.

There are many different methods of fasting, but all share the general goals mentioned above. Liquids taken during a fast may consist of water only, fruit juices, vegetable juices and broths, or herbal teas. Some physicians, like Andrew Weil, M.D., do not consider intake of any liquid except water or noncaloric herbal tea to constitute a fast. Although restricting one's intake to only broths or fruit or vegetable juices has its benefits, Dr. Weil believes such special dietary measures do not produce the same results as fasting.

Fasting can be short- or long-term. A short-term (one- to three-day) fast is often successful in the treatment of fever, cold, flu, digestive disorders, allergies, constipation, headaches, and rashes. It leaves many people feeling more alert and more energetic. Long-term fasts should be done only under expert supervision, as they can be dangerous. Long-term fasts have been credited with complete remission of diseases that have resisted other therapies; these conditions include bronchial asthma, ulcerative colitis, inflammatory disorders, and rheumatoid arthritis. Side effects of either form of fasting may include headache, bad breath, diarrhea, and vomiting.

Feldenkrais Method (FEL-den-kras) is an educational system that emphasizes how the body functions, the relationship between body movement and behavior, and how people learn behaviors. It is based on several concepts: everything people do, even thinking, involves movement; and, with proper training, people can teach their muscular and skeletal systems to hold and move the body optimally.

It was the contention of Moshe Feldenkrais (1904-84), the Israeli physicist who developed this movement therapy, that many postural problems, aches and pains, and in some cases skeletal muscle problems and distorted bone structure are the result of poor physical patterns learned in childhood or adulthood. The Feldenkrais Method offers instruction on how to relearn and reprogram body movements, which increases self-awareness of the physical state of being and the stresses placed upon it, and then gives them the tools to improve it.

The Feldenkrais Method consists of two parts. In the one-on-one portion of the program, called Functional Integration, teachers draw upon the approximately 1,000 different movements that make up the Feldenkrais Method to develop a program that is unique for each student and his or her needs and lifestyle. They use gentle touch to help realign posture, improve body movements, and help students become fully conscious of what is happening both internally and externally as they move. Feldenkrais teachers believe that once students are consciously aware of their movements, posture and balance will improve, chronic pains will disappear, and they will gain an overall sense of well-being.

The second part is Awareness Through Movement, during which students follow movements and exercises designed to increase their awareness of what the body is doing at all times. The simple exercises increase range of motion, improve coordination and flexibility, and, of course, augment body awareness.

The Feldenkrais Method can help people with lower back problems, arthritis, chronic pain, spinal pain, and postural problems. It also reportedly helps relieve symptoms of Parkinson's disease, multiple sclerosis, and cerebral palsy. ALSO SEE Alexander Technique

Feng Shui (fong shway) (Chinese for "wind and water") is a Chinese philosophy and an information system that focuses on the relationship between people and their environment, the subtle balancing and integration of their respective energies, and how these connections impact health and well-being. The principles of feng shui guide people on how to survive and succeed while living in harmony with nature by offering simple methods and steps to make their home, work, school, and social environments more harmonious. This may involve moving furniture, choosing new colors or wall coverings for a room or the house, adding plants, or changing the location of a picture or mirror.

Feng shui professionals help individuals custom-arrange their environments to fulfill their unique needs; therefore no two "prescriptions" are alike, even if two people ostensibly have similar lifestyles and physical surroundings.

Some aspects of feng shui, however, are universal and can be applied to all cases. For example, practitioners believe that the staircases in a home should not point directly at the front door, because beneficial **chi** can rush out the door. A feng shui professional would therefore recommend hanging a mirror on the back of the door that faces the steps.

Although new to Western ears and minds, feng shui has been practiced for more than 5,000 years and is rooted in the Taoist philosophy of nature, which includes the concept of **yin and yang**. It does not "cure" specific symptoms or ailments, but rather is a tool to achieve a state of well-being, balance, and harmony.

Fenugreek (FEN-yoo-grik) *(Trigonella graecum)* is a European herb whose dried ripe seeds have been used since ancient Egyptian times as a way to relieve sore throat pain and colds, and as an aphrodisiac.

It is believed fenugreek was first used as a food additive in spoiled feed for horses and cattle. The ancient Egyptians and Romans called the plant "Greek hay," which later became fenugreek. Soon, ancient physicians discovered the herb's mucilage (thick, sticky liquid) was useful in ointments to treat wounds and skin disorders. Ancient Chinese doctors used fenugreek to treat hernia, gallbladder conditions, impotence, and fever, while women in India found that the seeds increased their milk production while nursing.

Fenugreek has a taste similar to that of maple sugar, and in fact is widely used as a source of imitation maple flavor in the United States. Medicinally, fenugreek is often taken to help reduce blood sugar levels and the amount of harmful fats in the blood of people with insulin-dependent diabetes. Women who experience menopausal symptoms may get relief by adding fenugreek to their diets, as the seeds contain estrogenlike chemicals. The gelatinous substance called mucilage found in the seeds makes fenugreek effective in relieving constipation and diarrhea. External application of a fenugreek poultice (crushed fenugreek seed paste) can effectively treat inflammation and skin irritations and reduce the pain caused by neuralgia, swollen glands, and tumors.

Feverfew *(Tanacetum parthenium)* is an herb perhaps best known for its use in the treatment of headache, particularly migraine, and head pain associated with arthritis, fever, or inflammatory conditions. In ancient Greece and Rome, feverfew was prescribed for gynecological ailments. Its headache-relief abilities were noted in 1640 by British botanist John Parkinson and then about one hundred years later by English herbalist John Hill. Yet their discoveries were largely ignored except by practitioners of folk medicine. Interest in the herb was renewed in the 1980s in Britain after a woman who suffered with migraine followed the recommendation of a neighbor to chew feverfew leaves. The woman was the wife of a physician, and the success of her pain relief prompted him to urge study of the herb in the treatment of migraine pain.

Today many studies validate the herb's pain-relieving powers, including its ability to reduce inflammation and fever, soothe the digestive tract, and reduce blood pressure in some individuals. One reason for feverfew's ability to relieve head pain may be that it contains an ingredient called pathenolide, which inhibits release of **serotonin**, a neurotransmitter identified as a component in migraine. Other agents similar to pathenolide also appear in feverfew and are thought to help ease arthritis pain.

Feverfew is a perennial that sports daisylike flowers. It can be grown and maintained easily both indoors and out. ALSO SEE herbal medicine

Flavonoids (FLAY-vuh-noydz) (also called bioflavonoids) are powerful disease-fighting, **antioxidant** plant constituents found in various fruits, vegetables, herbs, and grains. They are sometimes referred to collectively as vitamin P. These often brightly colored compounds were discovered by Szent-Gyorgyi, the same scientist who discovered vitamin C.

Flavonoids have a long list of benefits, including that they protect against viruses and allergens; prevent heart disease, cancer, and blood glucose irregularities; strengthen and stabilize the cell membranes; and protect capillaries. Some of the most common flavonoids are hesperidin, quercetin, and rutin. All three of these flavonoids appear together naturally in citrus fruits. Rutin supplements are often derived from buckwheat while quercetin supplements are often made from algae. **Ginkgo** is a natural source of quercetin, while **green tea** is the source of another flavonoid, catechin.

There are many different flavonoids, some of which can be purchased as supplements either separately or combined with other nutrients. The federal government has not established an RDA (Recommended Daily Allowance) for flavonoids.

Flotation Therapy is a form of relaxation therapy in which individuals float in highly salted water that is enclosed in a flotation tank (general dimensions, 9 x 5 ft.) that allows in little or no external stimuli. Flotation tanks (also called isolation tanks) allow people to experience weightlessness in an environmentally controlled setting and to achieve a state of deep relaxation.

The idea for flotation tanks came from John Lilly, M.D., who was curious about the effect elimination of all sensory stimulation has on humans. Dr. Lilly and his colleague, Dr. Jay Shurley, introduced the first flotation tank in the 1970s. The theory is that sensory deprivation allows participants to connect with their inner thoughts and emotions and become motivated to make any necessary changes to their lifestyles. In some cases, tanks are equipped with speakers or videos that deliver music, meditation, or guided imagery instructions.

Flotation therapy may be useful in treating addiction, alcoholism, anxiety, smoking, insomnia, pain, tension, and stress-related disorders.

Flower Remedies are subtle mixtures of mineral water and the essence of flowers or trees, which many people claim can relieve mental and emotional distress and improve physical well-being. Perhaps the best known flower essence remedies are **Bach flower remedies**, which Dr. Edward Bach developed in the 1920s. His remedies stood alone until the mid-1970s, when a therapist named Richard Katz began to research new flower essences. Katz formed the Flower Essence Society, which has a database of more than 100 flower essences from more than 50 countries.

Flower remedies are made by floating fresh blooms in a bowl of spring water and leaving the bowl in sunlight on a cloudless day. This allows the essence of the flowers to "potentize" the water. Brandy is added to the potentized water to preserve the essence, and the remedy is stored in a dark glass bottle. Flower remedies are taken by adding a few drops of the essence into a small amount of mineral water and sipping the remedy slowly.

Most tree remedies are prepared in a similar way. One other method, created by French healer Patrice Bouchardon, involves dipping the buds, leaves, or blossoms of a tree into a salt solution to extract the essence. Sesame or sunflower seed oil is added to this mixture to preserve it. The tree remedy oils are massaged into specific parts of the body to promote self-healing.

Flower and tree remedies reportedly work at the body's energy level rather than at its chemical level and therefore are similar to homeopathic remedies. Treatment with flower and tree remedies work on the premise that emotional balance and harmony are necessary for good health, and these remedies are said to relieve negative emotions and moods and enhance well-being, which then allow the body's self-healing process to operate. Although there is no definitive proof of these claims, flower and tree remedies are used by many people to relieve nervous disorders, depression,

asthma, psoriasis, eczema, anxiety, chronic fatigue syndrome, and minor first aid problems.
ALSO SEE homeopathy

Fold and Hold is a natural pain-relief technique people can do for themselves, quickly and easily, and without the need for equipment. It is based on the fact that the body has a natural tendency to move from a position of pain or discomfort into one of comfort. This is demonstrated by the fact that children often sleep in what might be considered uncomfortable positions, yet their bodies have "found" the position naturally.

Fold and Hold was developed by an orthopedic surgeon, Dr. Dale L. Anderson, who studied how the body moves naturally to relieve pain as well as the effectiveness of "manmade" methods. The result of his research, Fold and Hold, is based on "nature's wisdom." Dr. Anderson estimates that 75 percent of common aches and pains can be reduced or eliminated using this method. The remaining 25 percent are caused by inflammation, infection, tumors, or trauma—which Fold and Hold is not designed to handle.

Fold and Hold is composed of four basic steps and consists of movements that are done slowly, gently, and within people's comfort zones. Fold and Hold relaxes and stretches muscles, which in turn relieves muscle spasm. Once pain is reduced or eliminated, other factors that may accompany the pain, such as tissue damage or swelling, can be addressed in a more relaxed, pain-free way. Back and neck pain are two of the most common ailments that respond well to Fold and Hold.

Folic Acid (or folate) is a member of the B-vitamin family and is essential for human health. It plays a key role in the maintenance and regulation of RNA and DNA and in the growth and function of all cells. When it was discovered in 1941, it was named after the Latin word *folium*, which means "leaf," because it was first extracted from spinach leaves.

The first use for folic acid was for the treatment of anemia. Subsequent research finds that women who take folic acid supplements are less likely to develop cervical cancer. Experts believe folic acid protects against cancer because a deficiency of folic acid causes changes in cell structure that are similar to those in the beginning stages of cancer. Folic acid, when combined with beta-carotene, is credited with reversing mild to moderate cervical dysplasia (abnormal tissue growth of the cervix).

Supplementation with folic acid is also found to reduce deaths from heart disease. It does this by decreasing the amount of homocysteine in the blood system—a substance that accumulates in the artery walls and places stress on the cardiovascular system. It also has been shown to prevent neural tube birth defects such as spinal bifida (incomplete closure of the neural tube around the spine) and anencephaly (incomplete or total lack of a brain), and therefore folic acid supplementation is now recommended for pregnant women and women of child-bearing age.

Deficiency of folic acid can cause irritability, apathy, hostility, and paranoid behavior, which can be corrected with increased intake of the vitamin. Symptoms of long-term deficiency of folic acid include graying hair, gastrointestinal disorders, impaired nutrient absorption, poor growth, and pernicious anemia. The best food sources of folic acid include brewer's yeast, spinach and other dark green leafy vegetables, orange juice, beets, and avocados.

GABA (Gamma-Amino-Buthyric-Acid) is a compound composed of amino acids that reduces electrical activity in the brain. It is most commonly used to reduce the severity of panic attacks and to induce sleep.

The human body produces GABA naturally; supplementation boosts the efficiency of the resident supply. There is some debate as to whether oral GABA produces a significant therapeutic effect. According to editors of the *National Panic/Anxiety Disorder Newsletter* (May-June 1994), GABA does not reach the brain when taken orally. Edmund Bourne, Ph.D., author of *The Anxiety and Phobia Workbook* and "Nutrition and Anxiety" in the *NPAD*, disagrees, stating that a small amount does penetrate the brain and produce a noticeable clinical benefit. GABA is available as an oral supplement and produces a calming effect without causing mental cloudiness.

Garlic *(Allium sativum)* is an odorous herb that has been used for a variety of ailments since at least 3000 B.C. It is a member of the allium family of vegetables, along with onions, shallots, and leeks. The ancient Egyptians were particularly fond of this herb and used it to relieve headache and sore throat. The ancient Greeks used garlic to treat snake and scorpion bites, ulcers, and gastrointestinal problems, while the Chinese and Japanese have been using it for centuries to lower high blood pressure. Army physicians used garlic juice during World War I to treat wounds and dysentery. We now know that garlic has strong antibiotic activity against many common bacteria.

According to James Duke, Ph.D., a botanist with the U.S. Department of Agriculture in Maryland, results of recent studies validate some of the above claims, and more. Garlic also helps protect against cancer of the stomach; reduces triglyceride and low-density lipoprotein cholesterol levels while increasing high-density lipoprotein cholesterol levels; decreases the possibility of the formation of blood clots that can cause heart attack; and helps eliminate lead and other toxic metals from the body. Some of garlic's medicinal benefits are attributed to one of its more than 200 compounds—allicin, a sulfur compound that acts as a powerful antibacterial agent and reduces blood clotting. Garlic also contains 32 other sulfur compounds, 17 **amino acids,**

vitamins A, B1, and C, as well as copper, calcium, **germanium**, iron, potassium, magnesium, **selenium**, and **zinc**. ALSO SEE herbal medicine

Geopathic Therapy (jee-o-PATH-ik) is a therapeutic approach in which practitioners attempt to identify sources of geopathic stress and then recommend how to avoid them. *Geopathic* stress is any negative energy that is emitted from the earth and from artificial sources, such as overhead power lines. Many experts believe prolonged exposure to geopathic stress compromises the immune system and thus makes the body susceptible to disease.

The effects of earth energies on health has long been recognized in Chinese culture. In the West, geopathic therapy is a more recent concept. To detect negative energy, practitioners use **dowsing** or **applied kinesiology**, or "sense" it as a physical sensation of energy in the body. One popular method of negating the effects of negative energy and restoring balance is **feng shui**, an ancient Chinese art that integrates people and their environments into a harmonious whole.

Proponents of geopathic therapy believe any health problem may be associated with negative energy and therefore recommend avoiding or eliminating exposure to negative energy sources such as power lines, microwaves, electric blankets, and electric appliances as much as possible. Geopathic therapy may be beneficial for headaches, migraine, sleep disorders, depression, anxiety and digestive disorders.

Gerda Alexander Eutony (GUR-duh YU-to-nee) (GAE) is a process that combines sensory-motor learning and mind-body awareness. The word "eutony" means well-balanced tension or tonicity, and this is the primary purpose of Gerda Alexander Eutony—to free up the tendency of muscles to remain contracted even when at rest and replace it with increased flexibility. According to Gerda Alexander (1908-93), who developed this technique, improved flexibility allows people to be more spontaneous and creative, both physically and emotionally as well as intellectually.

Instructors in GAE work with clients either one-on-one or in groups and teach them how to increase self-awareness, self-sensing, and self-knowing using various techniques, such as exploring the body in detail, stretching and noting how every muscle feels during the stretch, and focusing on where tension is hiding in the body. Every session is unique and tailored to the specific needs of the client, and it can benefit both able-bodied and physically challenged individuals.

Gerda Alexander Eutony is used in schools of dance and theater, by athletes and physical education departments, and by various commercial and medical organizations throughout Western Europe. In 1987, GAE was accepted by the World Health Organization as an alternative health-care method, the first mind-body technique embraced by the WHO.

Germanium (jer-MAY-nee-um) is a trace element that is found in the soil and in **aloe vera**, Siberian **ginseng**, **garlic**, **shiitake mushrooms**, **comfrey**, and sea algae. The naturally occurring mineral offers limited benefits to human health, but the synthetic version, most notably the one developed by the Japanese and called Ge-132 or Ge-Oxy 132, has significant medicinal value. The Japanese and others use Ge-132 to improve circulation and to help prevent cancer. It also appears to stimulate the body's immune system and to increase the production of a powerful anticancer, antiviral agent called gamma-interferon. Researchers are looking into the possibility that it will help fight AIDS, chronic fatigue syndrome, viral infections, and other immune-compromising conditions.

Gerson Therapy (or Gerson Diet) is a holistic, nutritional therapy that encourages the body's natural healing powers to fight chronic, degenerative illnesses. It was developed by Max Gerson, M.D. (1881-1959), who said,

"Stay close to nature and its eternal laws will protect you."
During his personal research of ways to cure himself of
migraine, he experimented with different foods and studied
the diets of apes. Soon he discovered that a diet of fruits,
greens, vegetables, and nuts cured not only his migraine
and those of other patients, it also was effective in the treatment of skin tuberculosis, arthritis, arteriosclerosis, diabetes, and other diseases. Gerson used his therapeutic
approach to treat his first cancer patient in the 1920s and,
after getting good results from other cancer patients,
brought Gerson therapy to the United States and published
his findings.

Gerson therapy seeks to regenerate the body by helping
it eliminate disease through the use of wholesome, simple
foods, juices, and nontoxic medications. The nutritional
plan is based on several primary features: restricted sodium
intake, potassium supplementation, extremely low fat intake, occasional temporary protein restriction, high intake
of **vitamins**, **minerals**, and micronutrients, and high consumption of fluids. Gerson believed that toxins interfere
with normal cell functioning and are the cause of disease.
Adherence to Gerson therapy allows the body to detoxify
and thus provides a healthy environment in which all cells
can function optimally.

Gerson therapy also usually involves biological medications, such as castor oil, pancreatic enzymes, and a liver
extract with vitamin B-12, and enemas of coffee or chamomile tea. The biological agents support optimal enzyme
activity and immune system functioning. The enemas remove toxins from the tissues and blood by stimulating the
enzyme systems in the stomach wall and liver and promoting the elimination of toxic bile.

According to the Gerson Institute, Gerson therapy "is
totally non-specific; by correcting the nutrition and helping
the body to detoxify, all the body systems can be reacti-
vated and restored, the metabolism is normalized and the
body can heal itself of chronic/degenerative disease."

Gestalt Therapy (guh-s(h)TALT) is a psychological therapy in which people learn how to increase self-awareness and acknowledge aspects of their personalities and feelings they have denied and repressed. "Gestalt" comes from a German word that means "meaningful whole." Thus Gestalt therapy is designed to help people know themselves better so they can more effectively and accurately interact with all segments of their environments.

Gestalt therapy was pioneered by Frederick S. Perls, Laura Perls, and Paul Goodman in the 1960s and gained popularity as an "active" therapy in which participants are permitted and encouraged to act out their feelings. This may take various forms, such as punching pillows, role playing, using puppets, or screaming. All behaviors are done in an emotionally safe environment to allow clients to explore and become comfortable with any new behaviors and feelings. Sessions may be one-on-one or consist of groups or workshops.

Gestalt therapy is most effective in resolving psychological issues such as depression and anxiety; however, it also can help improve stress and stress-related disorders and neurological problems, including insomnia and hyperactivity.

Ginger (*Zingiber officinale*) is a root herb found in many regions of the world. Ginger has been used in China for at least 2,500 years, where it is still valued as a digestive aid, a diuretic, and an antinausea/antivomiting agent. Scientists have now verified these uses and have uncovered even more. In Western societies ginger is especially valued in the treatment of nausea and upset stomach associated with motion sickness and morning sickness. Studies also show that ginger helps fight infections, lowers blood pressure and cholesterol levels, relieves earaches, reduces joint pain, and helps prevent blood clots. Certain chemicals present in ginger also may prevent the cell damage that is associated with cancer.

Ginger contains compounds called gingerols, which consist of volatile oil (evaporates easily) and resin. These agents appear to have some painkilling, anticough, and sedative properties. Ginger's ability to relieve or prevent nausea and vomiting is related to its direct action in the stomach and not to any impact on the central nervous system.

Ginkgo (GIN-ko) (*ginkgo biloba*; also called maidenhair tree) is the world's oldest surviving tree, and, for thousands of years, its leaves have been used by the Chinese to treat asthma. The roasted seeds were eaten by ancient Chinese and Japanese to aid digestion and prevent drunkenness. It has only been since the herb's introduction to Western medicine in the early 1970s that medical experts have discovered additional benefits, including its effectiveness in increasing blood flow to the brain, which helps people recovering from stroke; in improving memory; and in slowing the development of senile dementia and Alzheimer's disease. Ginkgo also helps reduce pain, treats ringing of the ears and chronic dizziness (vertigo), and relieves ·age-related vision loss (macular degeneration). Some studies even suggest it can relieve outbreaks of multiple sclerosis.

The extract of ginkgo leaves contains various active substances, called **flavonoids**, or ginkgogolides, which are believed to be responsible for ginkgo's ability to dilate (expand) the arteries and capillaries and thus increase blood supply and flow. Ginkgo extract is widely prescribed in Europe, including Germany, where it is dispensed for circulation disorders and asthma. In the United States, ginkgo is sold as a food supplement and is highly regarded for its potential to improve depression.

Ginseng (JIN-seng) (*Panax ginseng*; also *P. quinquefolius*, American ginseng; and *Eleutherococcus senticosus*, Siberian ginseng) literally means "root of man" and was so named because the ginseng root resembles the shape of the human body. The Chinese have used ginseng for more than 5,000 years and have prescribed it for hypertension, heart disease, poor blood circulation, and as an anti-aging agent. Because ginseng is an antioxidant, it helps the body eliminate harmful free radicals that contribute to the aging process.

Since ancient times, ginseng has been legendary as a tonic for longevity. Throughout ancient Asia, it became more precious than gold. When European missionaries visited Asia in the eighteenth century, they returned home with tales of its use. Jesuit missionaries to Canada in 1704 returned to Paris with samples of American ginseng, and soon interest was stirred on both sides of the Atlantic. American colonists soon lost interest, however, although some Native American tribes used the herb in love potions and to combat fatigue, aid digestion, and stimulate appetite.

A revived interest in ginseng in the United States did not occur until the 1960s, after I.I. Brekhman, Ph.D., a Soviet scientist, reported that Soviet soldiers who took ginseng extract could run faster than soldiers given a placebo. Dr. Brekhman's research led him to report that ginseng is an adaptogen, a substance that allows the body to better cope with stress and tension by enabling it to normalize body functions. Since then, various animal and human experiments have yielded many, sometimes conflicting, results. Ginseng reportedly can increase physical and mental performance, reduce cholesterol and triglyceride levels, alleviate menopausal symptoms, increase sexual desire, inhibit the growth of cancer cells, improve blood circulation, boost the immune system, and minimize the effects of radiation exposure.

Compared with other herbs, ginseng has an unusual number of constituents—more than 30—which has made it difficult to determine just how and why—and if—this herb has healing powers. The main active ingredients in ginseng are called ginsenosides; other compounds believed to have some healing effect include phenolic compounds and polysaccharides. To date, researchers are not certain how any of these ingredients act at the biochemical level in the body. It appears that ginseng affects the body's hormones. For example, ginseng seems to be beneficial in the treatment of stress, fatigue, high blood pressure, blood sugar levels, and sexual dysfunction—all of which are regulated by the hormones produced by the hypothalamus, adrenal glands, and pituitary gland.

Glucosamine Sulfate (gloo-KOH-suh-meen SUL-fate) is a compound that occurs naturally in all body tissues and is a vital component in holding tissue cells together. Glucosamine sulfate is also one of the chemicals that forms the major cushioning ingredients of the synovial fluids in the joints and surrounding tissues. These characteristics have led many individuals and some physicians to use glucosamine supplements to treat osteoarthritis.

As the body ages, it loses its ability to support healthy cell growth. Glucosamine sulfate supports the body's ability to supply the essential materials needed to replace old and worn-out cells and tissues. As a supplement, either alone or in combination with **chondroitin sulfate**, another sulfated sugar that occurs naturally in the body, it can be used to relieve the pain, stiffness, and inflammation characteristic of osteoarthritis. Chondroitin sulfate blocks the action of the enzymes that break down old cartilage.

The commercial supplements of glucosamine and chondroitin, which are extracted from crustacean shells (called chitin) and cow tracheas, have been used by veterinarians in the United States for many years for arthritic conditions in horses and dogs. In Europe, however, glucosamine has been used for people with osteoarthritis since 1980. One of the first reports was by Drs. Crolle and D'este, from the first Medical Division in Venice, Italy. Their research showed that glucosamine is as effective as painkilling drugs in reducing the pain associated with osteoarthritis, and the patients continued to improve even after treatment was stopped.

Osteoarthritis affects approximately 15.8 million Americans. The disease involves degradation, erosion, and loss of mechanical abilities in the joints, especially the knees, fingers, and hips, and is accompanied by pain and inflammation. Unlike conventional drugs, which merely treat symptoms and sometimes promote the disease process, glucosamine sulfate addresses the cause of osteoarthritis. It is credited with not only improving symptoms and in some cases eliminating them completely, but also with repairing damaged joints in some individuals.

Glucosamine and chondroitin sulfates are available in a combination compound called Cosamin®. This capsule reportedly can ''slow, halt or prevent the degeneration of cartilage,'' according to Jason Theodosakis, M.D., author of *The Arthritis Cure*. The Arthritis Foundation, however, warns that although some European studies suggest these nutrients are safe and effective in relieving pain, ''good, controlled, long-term studies are needed to see if the products are indeed helpful and safe,'' and to see whether they truly retard the degenerative disease process, says Doyt Conn, M.D., senior vice president of the foundation's medical affairs.

Glutathione (gloo-ta-THI-on) is a compound composed of three nonessential **amino acids**: cysteine, glutamic acid, and glycine. This combination, known as a tripeptide, is manufactured by the body and is also available as a synthetic supplement. Glutathione is found in all organisms on earth, and in humans it is most concentrated in the liver, spleen, kidneys, and pancreas. It performs several essential functions in humans, one of which is to help protect against a process called cross-linking of proteins, which can cause a decline in brain cell function. For this reason, glutathione is sometimes referred to as a ''smart nutrient.'' Glutathione is also important in guarding the stomach lining against hydrochloric acid and in protecting the body against environmental toxins, such as cigarette smoke, air pollution, and heavy metals.

Each of the three amino acids in glutathione performs specific duties. Cysteine helps protect against environmental toxins and prevents the oxidation of tissues that contributes to aging and cancer. Glutamic acid, the only amino acid metabolized by the brain, is involved in the metabolism of fats and sugars and produces **GABA**, which has a soothing effect on the brain. It is also used to reduce cravings for sweets and alcohol and to treat people with low blood sugar. Glycine stimulates production of glutathione, aids in detoxification, helps prevent stretch marks, and reduces sugar cravings.

Goldenseal *(Hydrastis canadensis)* (also known as yellowroot and puccoon root) is a perennial herb that grows throughout much of the United States. Though it was discovered by the aborigines of northern Australia, it was utilized extensively by the Cherokee and other Native Americans to treat skin infections, sore throat, recovery from childbirth, and digestive ailments. During the Civil War, goldenseal was used to treat wounds, and its success during that time prompted its continued use as an antibiotic. Researchers now know that goldenseal contains the powerful natural antibiotic called berberine, which kills many bacteria that cause diarrhea and may be effective against cholera bacteria, amoebic dysentery, and giardiasis.

Goldenseal also contains several alkaloids, which have mild antiseptic and astringent (drying) properties and which make it effective in treating conditions such as eczema and other skin disorders, cracked and bleeding lips, canker sores, and gum disease. The alkaloids also have a minor effect on the central nervous system, blood circulation, and uterine tone and contractility. When used as a douche, goldenseal can help relieve fungal infections. Goldenseal can also be used as a laxative and to relieve pain and irritation associated with hemorrhoids.

Goldenseal has been collected to near extinction and is now cultivated. Part of the problem with availability is that goldenseal is difficult to grow, and it takes five years for the roots to reach medicinal maturity.

Gotu Kola (GAH-too KO-lah) *(Centalla asiatica)* is an herb that grows well in moist or swampy areas in India, Sri Lanka, South Africa, and tropical areas of the United States. It probably originated in India in **Ayurvedic** herbal medicine treatment. There, gotu kola has been used as a mild diuretic and to treat skin inflammation. For approximately 2,000 years, the Chinese have used this herb to treat depression and other emotional problems associated with physical disorders. People in Sri Lanka believe the herb is an aphrodisiac and that it promotes longevity. This latter characteristic was assigned to gotu kola by people in Sri Lanka, who noticed that elephants, who have a long life-span, consume large amounts of this plant.

Gotu kola was used by Ayurvedic herbalists to treat problems of aging as well as skin diseases, especially leprosy. Today it is known that the chemical (asiaticoside) in gotu kola, which helps combat leprosy when applied to the skin, may be mildly carcinogenic. In the United States, gotu kola is used to improve memory, promote relaxation, and relieve anxiety and depression. Results of recent studies indicate that gotu kola strengthens the blood vessels and thus improves blood circulation, which makes it useful in the treatment of phlebitis, leg cramps, and other circulation problems. Gotu kola contains several glycosides known to have anti-inflammatory and wound healing abilities as well as a sedative effect. To date, no evidence has been found to substantiate claims that it promotes longevity.

Gravity Inversion Therapy (also called inversion therapy) uses the body's weight rather than physical weights or pulleys to provide traction. Children who hang upside down from the monkey bars at a playground are practicing gravity inversion therapy because they are allowing gravity to pull and stretch the top halves of their bodies.

When used as a means of treatment, gravity inversion can be accomplished in several ways. One way is to place your feet in special boots that are attached to an overhead bar and hang down; another is to strap yourself to a tilt table; and yet a third way is to hook your legs around the holding bar on a piece of gravity traction equipment.

Like other forms of **traction**, gravity inversion therapy can improve back pain by opening up the lumbar spine and relieving pressure on the discs. This technique has lost some of its following since the 1980s, when it was popular, although it can provide significant pain relief in many people. Adverse side effects can include an increase in blood pressure, headache, blurred vision, pressure behind the eyes, a stuffy nose, decreased heart rate, and retinal detachment.

Green Tea *(Camellia sinensis)* is the freshest and least processed form of tea. Like black tea, it is made from the leaves of the *C. sinensis* evergreen plant, but green tea retains the beneficial polyphenols that are removed when black tea leaves are fermented before drying. These polyphenols, in particular the **flavonoid** catechin, are reportedly responsible for the medical benefits attributed to green tea, one of which is a lower risk of cancer of the liver, pancreas, breast, lung, esophagus, and skin. Several studies of people with and without esophageal cancer, for example, show that those without cancer drank significantly more green tea than those with cancer. Green tea is also associated with lower risk of cardiovascular disease and stroke; reduced blood sugar levels; and ability to better fight off viruses.

Green tea has also been credited with helping people lose weight. This effect is believed to be caused by its caffeine content and by the fact that polyphenols and catechins promote the burning of fat. Suppliers of green tea do not agree on the amount of caffeine present in their products, as some claim green tea is naturally lower in caffeine than black tea while other researchers say the amount is similar.

Hakomi Integrative Somatics (ha-KO-mee) (or the Hakomi Method) is an integration of touch, **massage**, movement, energy work, and somatic awareness designed to help people establish an inner core of resources on which they can draw to heal the effects of traumatic and development injuries (injuries that progress over time, such as from overuse or to compensate for an imbalance). "Hakomi" is Hopi for "How do you stand in relation to these many realms?" with a modern translation of "Who are you?" Hakomi Integrative Somatics was developed by therapist and author Ron Kurtz in the mid-1970s and is based on the concept that the body and mind constantly interact and that the body reveals information about the unconscious mind. Thus a primary goal of the interaction between therapist and client is to build a relationship based on safety and partnership and one that promotes interaction between the conscious mind and the unconscious.

The Hakomi Method allows people to discover and study their mind-body patterns and core beliefs as they are experienced. This approach involves the use of **mindfulness**, a meditative practice of studying present experiences without judgment or effort. It also helps people change what Kurtz calls "core material"—the beliefs, memories, images, deep-seated emotions, and neural patterns people hold inside. Core material determines people's behaviors, attitudes, and perceptions and shapes them as individuals. Though some of this material is positive, some is also negative and serves to limit people physically, emotionally, mentally, and spiritually. The Hakomi Method helps clients distinguish between positive and negative core material and shows them how to effectively change anything that prevents them from growing as individuals.

The Hakomi Method draws from many influences, including Buddhism and **Taoism**—especially their concepts of gentleness, compassion, mindfulness, and respect for the wisdom of each individual. Hakomi also incorporates ideas from modern body-centered psychotherapies such as **bioenergetics**, the **Feldenkrais Method**, **Neuro-linguistic programming**, **Gestalt therapy**, and **Reichian therapy**.

Hanna Somatics (*somatics* means "self-controlling" or "self-sensing") is a systematic approach to sensorymotor education in which individuals who have disorders that affect their neuromuscular systems or who have chronically contracted muscles learn how to voluntarily control their muscles. It is sometimes referred to as a "cousin" of biofeedback because it allows people to control their own therapies.

Hanna somatics is based on the following concepts. All learning consists of both a movement and a sensory component. When people perform specific basic movements under controlled conditions, they experience sensations that help them identify tense areas in their muscular systems. Their movements stimulate the sensory and motor areas of the brain, and they learn to sense and move in those particular ways. As they continue to sense and move in new ways that eliminate tension, they gain smooth muscle control and relief from muscle spasticity.

Dr. Thomas Hanna, the creator of Hanna somatics, writes "that perhaps as many as fifty percent of the cases of chronic pain suffered by human beings are caused by sensory-motor amnesia (SMA)." Sensory-motor amnesia is the decline of sensory awareness and muscle control. The pain that accompanies SMA results primarily from chronic muscular contraction and fatigue. Secondary causes include compression of the joints and trapped nerves.

SMA is learned. It is the result of adaptive responses people make to injuries or stress, and the adaptation typically persists after the injury has healed. According to Hanna, these adaptations must be changed through sensory-motor learning—Hanna somatics.

Using specific movements designed by Dr. Hanna, people can, with practice, achieve significantly improved muscle control and coordination, reduced spasticity, pain relief, improved posture, increased flexibility, and better range of motion. They also learn to identify and correct other areas of excessive muscle tension as well as prevent additional ones from forming.

Proponents of Hanna somatics also believe that postural changes usually attributed to osteoporosis are, in most cases, caused by years of accumulated muscle tension. The same is true with the stiffness and pain generally blamed on aging. Hanna insists that older people are sore not because they are "old" but because their muscles are tight and overworked.

Hawthorn (*Crataegus oxycantha*) is a small thorny tree native to Europe that is considered by many herbalists to be the world's best heart tonic.

Hawthorn was not always known for its cardiac benefits. In ancient times, it was associated with fertility and marriage. Reports that Christ's crown of thorns was made of hawthorn caused this herb's positive reputation to become associated with death. It was used in the seventeenth century to treat kidney stones and finally was noted for its cardiac benefits by American settlers.

Today, however, hawthorn is used primarily in Europe, even though its value as a natural heart medication is acknowledged in the United States. Says Varro E. Tyler, Ph.D., professor of pharmacognosy at Purdue University School of Pharmacy in West Lafayette, Indiana, "hawthorn seems to have a direct positive action on the heart itself when taken over the long term. Apparently, it's a mild and harmless heart tonic." Most American physicians, however, warn people against self-medication with hawthorn for heart problems, especially if they are taking prescription medications.

Hawthorn dilates the peripheral and coronary blood vessels, increases the metabolism in the heart muscle, and improves blood supply to the heart. It can lower serum cholesterol, reduce blood pressure, and help prevent palpitations and arrhythmias. Its benefits to the heart are attributed to the fact that hawthorn is rich in **flavonoids**.

Hay Diet is a nutritional approach in which certain foods are combined in a specific way to maintain the proper balance of alkaline and acid mineral salts in the body. It was developed by Dr. William Hay, who acted on the research of Ivan Pavlov, a physiologist who discovered that meat eaten with starch takes twice as long to travel through an animal's stomach as does meat or starch eaten alone.

The Hay diet consists of three main food groups: alkaline-forming foods and two acid-forming food groups—concentrated carbohydrates and concentrated proteins. According to Hay, foods from the two acid-forming groups should never be eaten at the same meal, because each one requires a different digestive environment. Foods from either acid-forming group can be eaten with those from the alkaline-forming group, however, in a ratio of four times alkaline foods to one acid. This ratio ensures maintenance of the alkaline and acid mineral salt balance in the body. Hay also advocated allowing at least four hours between meals containing starch and protein. All refined or processed foods are prohibited, as are peas, beans, peanuts, and lentils. Starches, protein, and fats should be consumed in small quantities, while vegetables, fruit, and salad are emphasized. This dietary regimen reportedly has a significant effect on arthritis and digestive disorders and problems associated with obesity, such as hypertension and heart disease.

Hellerwork is a systematic series of **bodywork** treatment sessions that combines deep tissue manipulation, movement education, and interactive dialogue between client and therapist concerning emotional issues that emerge during sessions. Each of the eleven ninety-minute sections is structured to address specific body areas and functions. If the goals of a specific section are not reached within the ninety-minute time frame, the client will repeat the sections until desired results are accomplished. The program as a whole is designed to realign the body and release chronic stress and tension.

Hellerwork was developed in 1978 by Joseph Heller, who was the first president of the Rolf Institute and an aerospace engineer by trade. Heller studied **rolfing** and **Aston patterning** and formed his own opinions about and methods of **massage**, movement, and the mind-body connection. The concept behind Hellerwork is to provide a process by which people can improve their present "average" state of health to an optimal one, which Heller believes to be its natural state. People who seek Hellerwork often are experiencing pain and tension; however, Hellerwork focuses on rebalancing and realigning the body rather than on treating the symptoms of pain and tension. The result of realignment and rebalancing is pain relief, improved posture and alignment, better flexibility, and a more relaxed state.

Each Hellerwork section consists of three parts: bodywork, massage, and mind-body dialogue. During deep tissue manipulation, Hellerwork practitioners work on the fascia, a plastic-like tissue that surrounds the muscles and individual muscle fibers. Healthy fascia is moist and loose, but it becomes dry and rigid and forms knots when it is exposed to continual stress. Hellerwork practitioners release these knots using deep, connective tissue massage. Practitioners also help clients become intensely aware of the body and its movements and teach them new, easy ways to move with optimal alignment and balance. The dialogue portion of the program allows clients to become conscious of the relationship between the body and attitudes and emotions, which affects movement and self-expression.

Herbal Medicine is the use of plants for medicinal purposes. It has been practiced since recorded history, and probably before, and has existed in every culture throughout the world. For more than 4,000 years, plants used as medicines have been called "herbs" by Mediterranean and European cultures. In today's society, "herb" refers to any plant that is used for flavoring or medicine. When referring to herbal medicine, "herb" is any plant or plant part (flower, leaf, fruit, bark, root) that has medicinal and/or nutritional value.

Among the many types of herbal medicine systems in common use today, the most prevalent are the Chinese, **Ayurvedic**, European, Native American, and Western. All herbal systems share a common concept: the energy of plants is used to treat the body as a holistic unit, recognizing that each person has unique and changing needs. Among the systems, however, there are some differences in terminology, in how the herbs are gathered and prepared, and in how some of the herbs are prescribed.

Herbs are dispensed in many forms (see box), depending on the indication. Herbs are foods and, like any other food, should be taken in moderation. Herbalists, naturopaths, and others trained in the ways of herbs can help people decide which system and remedies are right for them.

Interest in herbal medicine systems is growing as more and more people become disenchanted with the ineffectiveness and toxicity of conventional drugs and seek a more natural, holistic, and economical approach to healing. An important principle of herbal medicine is that of "synergism," which asserts that the strength of the sum of the herb's parts is greater than the effectiveness of any individual parts. The belief is that nature created each herb as a finely orchestrated array of compounds, designed to work together. Each component has a distinct role in the healing process and in preventing adverse effects.

TYPES OF HERBAL FORMULAS

Herbs come in various forms and can be utilized in a wide range of ways. Below are some terms you may encounter while you investigate herbal remedies and preparations.

Pills, capsules, and powders are prepared herbs, available in natural food stores or pharmacies, from herbalists, or by mail order.

Infusions are made from the leaves, flowers, or other soft parts of a plant. They are prepared like teas, only they use more of the herb than other teas and they steep longer for greater potency.

Decoctions are prepared from the roots, stems, and bark of herbs. Because these plant parts are tougher than those used in infusions, decoctions need to steep longer than do infusions.

An **extract** is the juice obtained when the plant is crushed. Extracts are stronger than infusions and have a higher concentration of active ingredients.

Tinctures are extracts made with alcohol instead of water. They are usually made from potent herbs that are not suitable for infusions.

COMMONLY USED HERBS AND THEIR TREATMENT INDICATIONS

Aloe vera: burns, rash, wounds, and other skin conditions; hemorrhoids, and other skin conditions

Angelica: respiratory conditions, anemia, gynecological conditions

Bilberry: eye fatigue, glaucoma, day blindness

Black cohosh: menstrual cramps, pain of childbirth

Cayenne: arthritis, severe chronic pain, indigestion, infectious diarrhea

Chamomile: stress, diarrhea, indigestion, insomnia

Dandelion: menstrual symptoms, high blood pressure, congestive heart failure

Echinacea: colds and flu, bladder infections, skin disorders, candida

Elderberry: colds and flu, eczema, acne, psoriasis, nervous disorders

Ephedra: respiratory disorders, weight loss

Fenugreek: sore throat, colds, constipation, diarrhea, diabetes

Feverfew: headache and migraine, high blood pressure

Garlic: colds, flu, and bacterial infections; high blood pressure, wounds

Ginger: indigestion, nausea, high blood pressure, infections, earaches

Ginkgo: senile dementia and Alzheimer's disease, ringing in the ears, depression

Ginseng: high cholesterol, menopausal symptoms; boosts the immune system

Goldenseal: eczema and other skin disorders, gum disease, fungal infections

Gotu kola: skin conditions, stress, anxiety, depression

Hawthorn: heart disease

Kava: anxiety, muscle tension, pain

Lemon balm: nervous conditions, insomnia, headache, toothache

Licorice: respiratory conditions, hepatitis and cirrhosis, digestive disorders

Nettle:	hay fever, high blood pressure, gout, osteoarthritis
Peppermint:	indigestion, nausea, vomiting, diarrhea
Sage:	sore throat, canker sores, bleeding gums, diabetes
St. John's wort:	depression, anxiety, insomnia
Saw palmetto:	prostate enlargement, urinary disorders
Skullcap:	insomnia, headache, epilepsy, teething
Uva ursi:	urinary tract infections, yeast infections, painful menstruation
Valerian:	insomnia, stress, tension, anxiety
Wild yam:	menstruation, PMS, menopause

Holotropic Breathwork (ho-lo-TROP-ik) is a technique that combines rapid deep breathing, bodywork, and music as a way for people to open up the unconscious and unite body and mind in a state of altered consciousness. It is a highly experiential process that is usually performed in a group setting over a several-day workshop session.

Holotropic (meaning "moving toward wholeness") Breathwork was developed by Stanislav Grof, M.D., a psychiatrist and researcher of consciousness, and his wife, Christina. It is somewhat based on ancient yogic breathing methods. According to the Grofs, Holotropic Breathwork is not a therapy but "an adventure of self-discovery." They explain that all people have an inherent "radar" system that allows them to tap into whatever information they need to help them deal with or solve issues they have on their minds. To be most receptive to this information, the Grofs believe people need to engage in accelerated breathing—breathing faster and deeper than normal with no pauses in between (also known as circular breathing) while listening to loud, evocative music. This combination releases psychological defenses and allows unconscious or repressed thoughts and emotions to come forth. The breathing technique alone facilitates the release of toxins and reduces muscle tension.

Holotropic Breathwork may be beneficial for people who are seeking spiritual or emotional enrichment; those who have not had satisfactory results with long-term psychotherapy; or those who are experiencing stress-related disorders and pain.

Homeopathy (ho-mee-OP-uh-thee) is a holistic form of medicine in which the remedies given allow the body to heal itself. "Homeopathy" is a Greek word derived from *homios*, meaning "like," and *pathos*, meaning "suffering." Homeopathy, therefore, means treating "like with like." If you take a homeopathic remedy for nausea, for example, the substance is one that, if taken in a larger amount and by a well person, actually causes nausea. Homeopathic remedies, however, contain either a minute amount of a substance—or sometimes none at all except the essence of the substance—which effects a cure.

Homeopathy was founded by Samuel Hahnemann (1755-1843), a German physician and chemist who became disillusioned by conventional medicine and who experimented with different medicinal substances on himself and some of his colleagues. His work led him to make three general observations that are the pillars of homeopathy today. One is the law of similars, which says that a substance that can cause symptoms of illness or disease in a well person can, in minuscule amounts, eliminate those same or similar symptoms in someone who is ill. The second principle is that of minimum dose, which means that repeated dilution of a substance actually increases rather than decreases its curative powers and at the same time eliminates the risk of side effects. The third principle is prescribing for the individual. Because each person is unique and has his or her own specific needs, homeopaths (individuals trained to practice homeopathy) prescribe a remedy based on people's symptoms as well as on their physical and emotional states, temperaments, personalities, diets, lifestyles, and other characteristics that make them unique.

It is uncertain as to how homeopathy works, although countless studies have shown that it does. Homeopaths do note, however, that remedies work according to a set of three "rules" known as the "Laws of Cure": remedies begin to cure from the top of the head and work down; remedies work from the inside out and begin with major organs and go to minor ones; and symptoms disappear in reverse order of their appearance.

There are thousands of homeopathic remedies, but only about 200 are commonly prescribed. They can be used to treat a vast array of symptoms and conditions, from the common cold to cancer; from fear of public speaking to food poisoning; from back pain to indigestion.

COMMON HOMEOPATHIC REMEDIES AND THEIR TREATMENT INDICATIONS

REMEDY	SOME COMMON TREATMENT INDICATIONS
Aconite:	infections such as cold and flu; eye inflammation, asthma
Allium cepa:	cold and cough
Arnica:	bruises, pain or injuries associated with surgery, accidents, sports, dental work, and childbirth
Belladonna:	inflammatory conditions, flu, tonsillitis
Bryonia:	headache, rheumatism
Calendula:	wounds, burns, bleeding associated with dental extractions and childbirth
Euphrasia:	burning pressure in the eyes, headache with eye complaints, fever with chills

Hypericum:	injuries, wounds, tooth pain
Ignatia:	depression, eating disorders
Kali bichromicum:	nasal discharge, cough
Ledum:	puncture wounds, burns, stings, chronic joint pain
Natrum muriaticum:	headache associated with eyestrain or with chills and fever, mucus discharge that follows emotional trauma
Nux vomica:	indigestion, vomiting, diarrhea, constipation
Pulsatilla:	indigestion, menstrual cramps, morning sickness
Ruta:	muscle strains, fractures, eyestrain, rheumatism
Sepia:	menstrual and menopausal disorders, depression, backache, headache
Symphytum:	facilitates recovery from fractures, joint and cartilage trauma, and back and eye injuries

Hops *(Humulus lupulus)* is an herb that is well known both to herbalists and beer brewers. In herbal medicine, the entire plant is used for its ability to soothe the nerves, induce sleep, and calm anxious natures. To treat these conditions, herbalists may prescribe a tea or sleeping with a pillow stuffed with hops and lavender. Hops also has pain-killing properties and is useful in the treatment of toothache, neuralgia, headache, and earache. Hops can be applied externally as a poultice and used to treat inflammation, sores, boils, rashes, and cysts. A resinous dust called lupulin, found in the plant's fruit, is responsible for most of the plant's medicinal value.

Humor Therapy is the use of humorous stimulation—literature, jokes, movies, videos, and so on—to combat stress, stress-related physical ailments, and other health problems. Laughing boosts the immune system and triggers production of beta-endorphins, the body's own natural, morphinelike, pleasure-inducing chemicals in the brain. According to Dr. Lee Berk, professor of pathology and laboratory medicine at Loma Linda University in California, "If we took what we now know about laughter and bottled it, it would require FDA approval."

Dr. Berk and others have shown that laughing reduces blood pressure, increases muscle flexion, and boosts production of natural killer cells (which destroy viruses and tumors), gamma-interferon (a disease-fighting protein), B-cells (which produce disease-destroying antibodies), and T-cells (which are important in the immune system). Laughter also helps stop the flow of stress hormones, which not only cause blood pressure to rise but also increase the number of platelets in the blood, which can cause obstructed arteries and heart attack. Regular bouts of laughter, therefore, are believed to be preventive as well as therapeutic.

The importance of humor in healing has been endorsed by the American Association for Therapeutic Humor. Research into the effects of humor on health continues, including studies of the impact on the immune system of people with cancer and AIDS.

Hydrogen Peroxide Therapy is a form of **oxygen therapy** in which medical grade hydrogen peroxide is used to treat health problems. Hydrogen peroxide (H_2O_2) is water with an extra atom of oxygen.

Hydrogen peroxide comes in various strengths; a 35 percent solution, also known as food-grade hydrogen peroxide, is the strength used for medicinal purposes. It is called food-grade because it is used in food products such as cheese, whey products, and eggs. When used for healing, it can be applied topically to the skin or taken internally. For treatment of skin conditions such as rash, eczema, herpes, cuts, abrasions, and other problems, patients can bathe in a diluted hydrogen peroxide solution or spray a diluted solution on the body after a hot shower. For conditions such as candida, gastrointestinal problems, gynecological infections, diabetes, HIV-related problems, and Epstein-Barr virus, physicians can administer intravenous injections of diluted hydrogen peroxide. It also can be taken orally.

Hydrogen peroxide therapy boosts the body's immune system and its ability to fight viruses, bacteria, and other pathogens. It also increases the delivery of oxygen to the cells and stimulates cellular respiration.

Hydrotherapy (also called water therapy) is a broad term for the therapeutic use of water. Water therapy can take many forms, and includes but is not limited to soaking in hot springs or spas, exercising in the water, use of steam vapors, and alternating hot and cold showers.

Hydrotherapy, or "taking the cure" as it was often referred to in the eighteenth and nineteenth centuries, has existed in some form for millennia. The first hydrotherapy treatments likely consisted of bathing in mineral springs. In Europe, spas evolved around the use of hot, warm, and cold springs, and elaborate buildings were erected to house them. These spas are still popular today.

Naturopaths are the practitioners who most often prescribe hydrotherapy; however, physical therapists, osteopaths, and some bodywork therapists incorporate various hydrotherapy techniques when appropriate. Hydrotherapy is prescribed to improve blood circulation, reduce fever, cleanse the bowels, stimulate the flow of vital energy, and relieve tension. Taking alternating hot and cold showers, for example, stimulates blood and lymph circulation, relieves lung and nasal congestion, and tones the skin and tissues. To relieve constipation and piles or to treat liver or kidney problems, a similar concept called sitz baths is used. In sitz baths, patients sit in a bowl of hot water and place their feet in a bowl of cold, and vice versa. Respiratory problems and sore throat are often treated with inhalation of steam, while impacted feces and toxic bowel (bowel infected with harmful bacteria) are remedied with enemas. Application of hot or cold water compresses is a common treatment for painful or inflamed joints and bruises. Other forms of hydrotherapy include steam baths, Turkish baths, sitting in a sauna, and soaking in a whirlpool.

In addition to the conditions mentioned above, hydrotherapy is used for acne, anemia, arthritis, asthma, back pain, bruises, hypertension, bronchitis, chronic fatigue syndrome, colitis, cramps, depression, hemorrhoids, gout, gallstones, fluid retention, irritable bowel syndrome, menstrual problems, migraine, muscle weakness, nervous disorders, neuralgia, sleep disorders, stress, tension, ulcers, vertigo, and wheezing.

ALSO SEE colon hydrotherapy

Hyperbaric Oxygenation Therapy (hi-per-BA-rik) is a noninvasive therapeutic method that involves exposing people to an environment of 100 percent oxygen at an atmospheric pressure greater than normal (*hyper* means "high"; *baric* means "atmospheric pressure"). This therapy is used to treat people who have a disease or an injury that results in a decreased or insufficient supply of oxygen to any part of the body. It is growing in popularity for treatment of circulation problems, diabetes, heart disease, multiple sclerosis, gangrene, and stroke, and in difficult-to-treat conditions, such as foot ulcers, burns, and bone infections. Hyperbaric oxygenation therapy is one of three kinds of oxygen therapy; the other two are **ozone therapy** and **hydrogen peroxide therapy**.

The air we normally breathe contains 21 percent oxygen, which is usually sufficient for the body to heal. To facilitate poor circulation or to treat hard-to-resolve conditions, such as a diabetic skin ulcer, in which the white blood cells need 20 times more oxygen to fight and kill the bacteria associated with the wound, hyperbaric oxygenation therapy is an option. Treatment takes place in a sealed chamber in which the patient sits or reclines as oxygen is either pumped in and allowed to surround the entire body or is introduced through a mask or head tent. In either case, the oxygen the patient breathes is absorbed in the body by the blood. After a treatment, oxygen levels remain elevated in the tissues for several hours. In this enriched environment, new capillaries grow and help provide more blood to the injured or compromised site. Hyperbaric treatment also makes red blood cells more flexible so they flow more easily through the capillaries.

Hyperbaric oxygen therapy was developed in the late 1800s to treat decompression sickness (''the bends'') in deep-sea divers who returned to the surface too quickly. Today there are about 260 hyperbaric oxygen therapy facilities in the United States.

Hypericum (hi-PER-ih-cum) *(Hypericum perforatum)* is the traditional name for the homeopathic remedy known as **St. John's wort**, in herbal medicine. In **homeopathy**, hypericum is used primarily as a first aid remedy for injuries to sites that are rich in nerves, such as the fingers, lips, nails, and spine. For example, an injury to the hands or a blow to the head that sends shooting pain along the nerve path responds well to hypericum. This remedy is also indicated for use after a lumbar puncture or spinal injection, tooth pain, gaping wounds that involve nerve damage, and old scars that are still painful. Generally, pain is worse for pressure and movement and better for lying on the painful site. The typical hypericum personality is one of deep depression associated with an injury involving the nerves.

Hypnotherapy is the therapeutic use of hypnosis, a heightened, altered state of consciousness in which individuals are awake but intently focused, as if in a trance. During a hypnotic state, people are deeply relaxed but always in control. They openly accept and respond to suggestions, yet they will not do or say things that go against their principles. All five senses become more acute.

Hypnotherapy was practiced in ancient Greece, where

priests and healers used it to treat both physical and emotional disorders. Modern hypnosis is generally credited to the Austrian Anton Mesmer who, in the eighteenth century, tried to harness mental energy. His attempts resulted in his "mesmerizing" his clients and attracting the attention of Dr. James Braid, who coined the word "hypnosis." Subsequent investigations have proved hypnotherapy to be effective in the relief of pain and the alleviation of stress, tension, and anxiety. It is taught in many medical schools and has been approved by the American Medical Association since 1958.

Hypnosis is used by mental health practitioners; by dentists to help patients overcome the fear of dentists and dental procedures; and by various therapists to help people lose weight, quit smoking, eliminate phobias, and other goals. Ninety-four percent of people who undergo hypnotherapy receive some benefit from it, even if it is only relaxation.

Hypnotherapy is generally used in three ways: to help people examine and analyze the roots of their particular problems; to eliminate physical, emotional, and mental tension; and to replace negative thoughts with positive ones. These goals can be reached while working one-on-one with a hypnotherapist or by learning self-hypnosis techniques from a professional. Hypnotherapists can use many different techniques to achieve a client's desired goal once the mind is focused; some of them include: distraction, reprogramming to less painful ways of thinking, substituting another physical response to stress, processing causes of stress to find alternatives in your life, and uncovering old emotions.

Because hypnotherapy allows access to the unconscious mind, the situations for which it can be effective are varied. They include but are not limited to stress- and anxiety-related conditions, such as phobias, panic attacks, lack of self-esteem and self-confidence, stuttering, headache, impotence, irritable bowel syndrome, and dermatitis; addiction to drugs, alcohol, nicotine, and gambling; and depression, aggression, listlessness, and other mood disorders.

I

Ideokinesis is a word created from the Greek *ideo*, which means "idea," and *kinesis*, which means "motion." Ideokinesis is a technique to reeducate the neuromuscular system by using mental imagery to alter movement patterns.

Lulu E. Sweigard, Ph.D., created ideokinesis based on her work as a dance teacher. The focus of her technique is the idea that the nervous system is responsible for coordinating all musculoskeletal movement and postures; therefore, people who want to change their postures or how they move must first consciously change their neurological activity. Sweigard also believed that many of the aches and pains people experience are the result of an imbalance in muscle strength and how they use their muscles. To correct this she asked people to picture "lines of movement" traveling throughout the body and then used this concept to help them balance their muscle activity and centers of gravity. This approach allows people to teach or train their nervous systems to stimulate or move muscles in a proper, more balanced way.

Ideokinesis is a nonstrenuous tool that allows people to reeducate their muscles and movement patterns. Sweigard stressed that people need to have an understanding of anatomy and biomechanics in order for the technique to work well. Dr. Sweigard did not establish a school or formally train teachers in her technique; however, many individuals who teach dance or movement use ideokinesis.

Ignatia (ig-NAY-shee-uh) *(Ignatia amara)* is a homeopathic remedy made from the seed pods of St. Ignatius's bean *(Strychnos ignatia)*, which contain strychnine. In homeopathic doses, the amount of this poison is so minute it does not cause problems. Ignatia is indicated for a variety of emotional conditions, especially recent depression associated with grief and loss, as well as eating disorders such as bulimia and anorexia, which usually have strong emotional undertones. Other symptoms that indicate ignatia may include an insatiable appetite for raw food, yawning and sighing, insomnia, bad dreams, sleepwalking, and the sensation of a lump in the throat.

The ignatia personality includes people who are emotionally sensitive and unpredictable: they may laugh hysterically, sob uncontrollably, or suddenly throw a tantrum. Their extreme emotional states can cause them to develop nervous headaches, facial tics, muscle spasms, and numbness.
ALSO SEE homeopathy

Imagery (IM-aj-ree) is a process that involves visualizing objects, scenes, or other images in the mind's eye and then using what is seen to send healing messages to the body. This form of mind-body medicine is advocated by many physicians and researchers who have seen it work in healing ailments as diverse as bed sores, high blood pressure, acne, arthritis, stress-related conditions, chronic pain, and cancer.

A great deal of mystery surrounds how imagery works, and several hypotheses address this question. One is that people have the ability to consciously cause their immune systems to work on and heal weak sites in the body. Some people with cancer, for example, have reportedly "imagined away" their cancer cells. Another suggestion is that because so many physical ailments are directly associated with the mind-set—that is, brought on by stress and anxiety in people's lives—that focused imagery involving stress-relieving scenes or circumstances is enough to dispel many physical and psychological conditions. Finally, the simple yet powerful conviction that imagery will work may be all people need to experience relief.

Imagery sessions are often guided, which means people explore one or more images with the help of an audiotape, a book, or with a therapist. A typical therapeutic session begins with a relaxation exercise, which allows the individual to focus his or her attention. Some people find that hypnosis helps them center themselves. (Hypnosis is not the same as imagery. The former is a state of mind while the latter is an activity.) During the imagery portion of the session, the client is immersed in the image(s) he or she has called upon to help resolve a particular problem or ailment. These images may involve visualization as well as the other senses—smell, taste, hearing, and touch.

An advanced technique called positron emission tomography (PET), which can detect and display where activity is occurring in the brain, has shown that the same part of the brain is activated regardless of whether people actually experience something or whether they just imagine it. The more vivid a person's imagination and the more senses he or she brings to an imagery session, the more likely the session will effect the desired change. Imagery is a valuable mind-body tool because it can result in physiological change, help people deal better emotionally with their illnesses, and reveal any connection between their physical symptoms and the stress in their lives. In addition to the conditions named above, imagery can affect the body's need for any medications a person may be taking.
ALSO SEE hypnotherapy

Inositol (in-OH-sih-tol) is a vitamin-like substance that is present in the cell membranes in the form of phosphatidylinositol. It is manufactured in the body, particularly by the bacteria in the intestines, and it assists in nerve transmission, regulation of enzyme activity, and helps in the mediation of cellular response to external stimuli.

In the late 1970s, scientists discovered that people who were depressed had lower levels of inositol in their spinal fluid than people who were not. Nearly 20 years later, studies conducted at Israel's Ben Gurion University indicated that inositol is effective in the treatment of depression and panic disorder.

Although no Recommended Daily Allowance (RDA) has been established for inositol, it is believed that a deficiency may lead to diabetes. Supplementation may prevent, correct deficiencies caused by, or help alleviate problems with blood glucose levels in people with diabetes. Inositol is found in the seeds and leaves of most plants, and major food sources include whole grains, legumes, vegetables, and nuts.

Iridology (ir-ih-DOL-o-jee), or "iris diagnosis," is a scientific diagnostic technique that involves studying and analyzing the iris (the color portion of the eye) to discover information about tissue changes and areas of inflammation in the body. Iridology was developed by Ignatz von Peczely, a physician who noted a relationship between tissue changes in the body and markings on the iris. During his research he developed the first iridology chart, which has since been revised numerous times.

The iris contains hundreds of thousands of nerve endings that, through the nervous system, are intimately connected to every tissue in the body. Signals of pain, inflammation, or other conditions are transmitted along the nerve fibers and picked up by the endings in the iris, which then reveals the body's strengths, weaknesses, and general state of health. Iridologists, who are trained to read the more than 180 zones that have been mapped out on iridology charts, can then detect areas of strength, weakness, injury, or degeneration in the body by "reading" the patterns, color variations, structures, and degrees of lightness and darkness in the iris. An iridology reading can detect chemical and nutritional imbalances and accumulated toxins, as well as areas that are healing. It can serve as an early warning system, indicating problem areas before symptoms appear. It cannot identify a specific disease or locate viruses and other germs, but it can indicate any inflammation or other toxic condition they may be causing.

Some iridologists practice nutrition therapy and herbal medicine and may recommend specific herbs or supplements for conditions they diagnose.

Jin Shin Do (GIN shin doo) (also called jin shin do bodymind acupressure) is an acupressure technique combining traditional Japanese acupressure methods, Western psychology, and **Taoist** philosophy and breathing techniques. Jin shin do means ''The Way of the Compassionate Spirit'' or ''The Way of the Heart'' and is a complete mind-body therapy that relieves pain and both physical and emotional stress and tensions.

Jin shin do works on the principle that the body has energy fields or reservoirs called extraordinary vessels, which are more primal than the twelve **meridians** referred to in Oriental medicine and therapy. Practitioners of jin shin do believe the extraordinary vessels and organ meridians work together and that the vessels help compensate for any energy imbalances in the meridians. Therefore, jin shin do is often recommended as treatment for situations that have not responded well to meridian balance techniques, such as endocrine and hormonal problems, chronic disease, severe fatigue, and metabolic disorders.

Jin shin do differs from **shiatsu** in that it focuses more on deep release of tension. It also differs from traditional **acupressure** because it works more on a spiritual level and is a way for the recipient to connect with his or her own adventurous and compassionate inner spirit. Jin shin do is often referred to as a shared experience because the practitioner does not "do" a treatment inasmuch as he or she shares the experience with the recipient.

Iona Marsaa Teeguarden developed jin shin do as she studied with masters of various bodywork techniques in the United States and Japan. People can receive treatments from a professional jin shin do practitioner or learn how to treat themselves and others by using the 30-point system, methods of release, and color chart formulated by Teeguarden.

Conditions that often respond well to jin shin do include headache, back and neck pain, insomnia, eyestrain, fatigue, tension, anxiety, depression, guilt, anger, colds, fibromyalgia, lack of motivation, premenstrual syndrome, and foggy thinking. It also restores balance and promotes deep relaxation, inner peace, and raised awareness.

Jin Shin Jyutsu (gin shin gee-YOOT-soo) is an ancient Japanese art of releasing tensions that are stored in the body. Practitioners and teachers emphasize that jin shin jyutsu is an "art" rather than a "technique" because this approach is a skilled creation rather than a mechanical function.

The literal translation of *jin shin jyutsu* is "art of the Creator through man of knowing and compassion." It was practiced before the birth of Gautama Buddha and Moses, but because the art was passed on orally, it all but disappeared until the early 1900s when a Japanese shaman taught a philosopher named Jiro Murai, who was very ill at the time, some of the hand techniques. After Murai recovered, he conducted extensive research of jin shin jyutsu and eventually incorporated knowledge of acupuncture into it.

Jin shin jyutsu practitioners promote the flow of vital energy throughout the body and help release any blockages by placing their hands on two different points of the 26 on the body that have been identified as "safety energy locks." As they apply gentle pressure, practitioners act as a channel through which energy flows, recharging the recipient's body and unblocking "stuck" energy. In this way jin shin jyutsu is like **acupuncture** in that it facilitates the flow of **chi**. Practitioners of jin shin jyutsu use an energy map of the body, which is similar to the acupuncture **meridian** map, but containing only 26 points.

Jin shin jyutsu was introduced to the United States by Mary Ino Burmeister, who studied extensively with Murai. Mary insists that jin shin jyutsu is an inborn ability that everyone can learn and apply to heal oneself or others. ALSO SEE acupuncture

Kali Bichromicum, or potassium bichromate, is a homeopathic remedy that is prepared from the bichromate of potash, which derives from chromium iron ore. The most characteristic symptom for this remedy is excessive mucus discharges from mucous membranes anywhere in the body, especially the nose and throat. Nasal discharge is chronic and may be accompanied by headache. Localized, severe pain that appears suddenly and affects areas about the size of a dime and then disappears rapidly is another common characteristic. If there is cough, it is worse in damp, cold weather and may be better when lying down in a warm bed.

Individuals who benefit from kali bichromicum are usually listless, averse to physical and mental exertion, intolerant of carbohydrates, and distrustful of strangers. ALSO SEE homeopathy

Kava *(Piper methysticum)* is a perennial shrub that belongs to the pepper family. Anthropological evidence indicates that it has been cultivated and used for more than 3,000 years by various societies in the South Pacific. It is still used there today for spiritual, recreational, and medicinal purposes.

Kava is valued for its muscle relaxing, antianxiety, anesthetic, and analgesic effects. Scientific analyses show that the compounds responsible for these properties, called kavalactones, are located in the plant's roots. Other studies suggest that kava is also an anticonvulsant and a diuretic, decongestant, antiseptic, antifungal, and antibacterial agent.

Kinetic Awareness Therapy, also known as "ball work" because balls are used as part of the therapy, is a method of body reeducation. It allows participants to release inappropriate tension and enables them to work with and use appropriate tension in the body.

Kinetic Awareness was created by Elaine Summers, a dancer and choreographer who was told at the age of twenty-seven that her osteoarthritis would cripple her in five years. She fought back by studying **Sensory Awareness therapy** and combining it with her knowledge of dance and movement. The result was Kinetic Awareness.

Summers maintains that the body holds "frozen tension," tension held unconsciously and chronically until posture, movement, and alignment are adversely affected. During Kinetic Awareness sessions, participants use various sizes of rubber balls to help them focus attention on areas that are tense and then massage and stretch those areas by moving their bodies over the balls.

Kinetic Awareness is taught in five phases, which are cumulative. Practitioners teach clients anatomy, how to move each body part separately, awareness of total body systems, breathing, and how to change tension levels consciously. Once participants complete the five phases (each phase is more than one session), they can use the technique at any time on their own. Kinetic Awareness is useful for dancers, athletes, and other performers, as well as anyone who wants to increase flexibility, range of motion, coordination, and energy levels. It is also effective for dealing with chronic pain and recovering after injuries.

Kirlian Photography (KER-lee-en) is a diagnostic technique in which special photographs are taken of a living organism—in people it's usually a photograph of their hands—to reveal the energy radiations it is emitting. A trained practitioner then can interpret the various flares and diminished areas of energy in the photographs to help identify areas of strength and imbalance in the body. Kirlian photography is strictly a diagnostic tool and not a method of treatment.

Kombucha (kom-BOO-cha) is an ancient healing food and tea that originated in Asia and was a popular healing remedy in the 1920s and 1930s in Russia, Austria, Germany, and Czechoslovakia. It was introduced into the United States in the late 1980s and quickly gained a reputation as a "miracle" healing beverage for an extensive list of symptoms, ailments, and conditions.

Although widely referred to as a mushroom, kombucha is actually a combination of yeast and bacteria. Herbalist Pastor Weidinger, a missionary in Taiwan, was introduced to the tea and its history. Called "K'un Puch'a" among the natives, it was originally prescribed by a Korean medicine man named Kom-bu in the year 414 for the Japanese emperor's health problems.

Weidinger describes kombucha as a lichen, a plant organism that is "a symbiosis of algae and fungi." It is composed of several tropical yeasts and a few bacteria, the most important of which is the slimy vinegar bacteria *Acetobacter xylinum*.

According to Dr. Rudolf Sklenar, who conducted extensive experiments with kombucha, he has successfully treated diabetes, hypertension, digestive ailments, stomach and bowel diseases, rheumatism, and gout. He published his findings in the 1960s, and worldwide interest was piqued. Nobel Prize winner Aleksandr Solzhenitsyn reportedly fully recovered from cancer after taking kombucha, and his success prompted former president Ronald Reagan to take kombucha daily, while in office, for his cancer.

Kombucha tea is prepared using a kombucha culture and a specific formula of tea, water, sugar, and vinegar (original batch only). The combination sets off a fermentation process that produces various acids, enzymes, and vitamins. Among the acids are usinic acid, an antibacterial and antiviral agent, and lactic acid, which detoxifies, purifies, and strengthens the body.

Proponents of kombucha claim it can cure a long list of diseases and conditions, including but not limited to osteoarthritis, constipation, back pain, chicken pox, shingles, abscesses, cataracts, hypertension, heart disease, cataracts, diarrhea, sleeping disorders, cancer, and hemorrhoids. It also reportedly lengthens lifespan, cleanses the blood, eases symptoms of HIV and AIDS, increases energy levels, boosts the immune system, eases symptoms of chronic fatigue syndrome, prevents cancer, restores visual acuity, prevents menopausal symptoms, reduces the formation of wrinkles, enhances libido, reduces the risk of gallstones and liver problems, helps restore color to gray hair, improves baldness, strengthens the kidneys, strengthens the leg muscles, and reduces obesity.

To date, reports of kombucha's healing powers are anecdotal and yet to be proven in clinical trials.

Lavender (*Lavandula officinalis*, and other species) is a flowering plant whose essential oil is one of the most commonly used by aromatherapists, herbalists, naturopaths, and other natural health practitioners. Lavender is best known for its sedative and antidepressant properties. When the vapors are inhaled or the oil is massaged into the skin, it is effective for the treatment of anxiety, insomnia, nervous tension, migraine, and headache caused by tension or associated with cold and flu. It can encourage the passage of gas, ease muscle spasms, promote restful sleep, and increase blood circulation. When made into a tea, it is used to prevent fainting and to relieve nausea. Lavender also is an antiseptic and is useful in the treatment of wounds. Indeed, it was lavender's wound-healing abilities that prompted the resurgence of **aromatherapy**.

Lecithin (LES-ith-in) see choline

Ledum *(Ledum palustre)* is a homeopathic remedy derived from a small shrub known as wild rosemary. The entire fresh plant or just the twigs can be used to prepare the remedy. Ledum is valued both as a first aid remedy for injuries such as puncture wounds, bites and stings, and blows to the eye, and for chronic conditions that involve joint pain, such as rheumatism. Symptoms that signal use of ledum include extreme thirst for cold water, pain that is better for cold and worse for warmth, feeling chilled and cold to the touch, and bad dreams. Individuals best suited for ledum are described as being somewhat discontented and full of self-pity.
ALSO SEE homeopathy

Lemon Balm *(Melissa officinalis)*, also known as sweet balm and melissa, is so named because it has a distinct lemony taste. Lemon balm is a member of the mint family, and the botanical name *Melissa* is derived from a Greek word meaning "honey." The ancient Greeks placed lemon balm in beehives to attract bees.

Traditionally, lemon balm has been used to treat nervous problems, insomnia, headache, toothache, menstrual cramps, tumors, and insect bites, and these uses continue today. More recently, it has gained attention as a treatment for hyperactive children. Studies conducted in Europe have revealed that lemon balm has strong antiviral action against herpes virus when applied topically.

Licorice *(Glycyrrhiza glabra)* is a controversial herb that has been used for thousands of years as a treatment for colds, arthritis, hepatitis, cough, ulcers, and infection. Critics of its use say it has dangerous side effects, which can be avoided if the herb is taken with caution.

Licorice has been a popular healing herb among the Chinese for nearly 5,000 years, who used it to treat cough, malaria, food poisoning, liver problems, and some cancers. References to licorice are abundant throughout history, from ancient Greece to seventeenth-century England. American settlers found the Native Americans drinking licorice tea as a laxative and cough remedy. Contemporary herbalists recommend licorice for respiratory problems, digestive disorders, and liver problems such as hepatitis and cirrhosis. Licorice's anti-inflammatory properties make it useful in treating arthritis, and its antiviral abilities are useful in treating herpes sores, yeast infections, and wounds when sprinkled on in powder form. Scientists attribute licorice's healing abilities to a chemical called glycyrrhetinic acid.

Light Therapy (also called phototherapy) involves exposure to sunlight or sun-like light (also called natural lighting or full spectrum lighting) as a way to treat various forms of depression, the "blues," seasonal affective disorder (SAD; severe winter depression), and other related conditions. Researchers have found that reduced sunlight hours in the winter cause many people to feel moderately to severely depressed, out of sorts, abnormally tired, drowsy during the day, anxious, hopeless, and socially withdrawn. In many cases, prescribed daily exposure to high-intensity artificial sunlight is one way to eliminate these symptoms. The use of bright light therapy suppresses the secretion of melatonin, a hormone naturally produced by the brain and only released at night—or when it is dark. The bright light also appears to increase the effectiveness of **serotonin** and other neurotransmitters, which helps keep mood elevated. Thus light therapy appears to be the only effective way to influence circadian rhythms.

Exposure to bright light can come from overhead fluorescent tubes (eight four-foot bulbs emit 10,000 lux, the standard for measuring light intensity) or from a light box that sits on a table. Other ways to increase exposure to light during the winter months include making a conscious effort to go outside during the day, sitting near a window when possible, and taking a vacation to a sunny destination.

Light therapy can relieve depression and "feeling blue," reduce the effects of jet lag, shorten very long menstrual periods, and treat insomnia, eating disorders, and psoriasis. It also reportedly can reduce symptoms of lupus.

Lomilomi Massage (LO-mee-LO-mee), which literally means "rub rub" in Hawaiian, is an ancient massage technique that involves special finger movements that break up muscle spasms throughout the body. The relaxing yet highly revitalizing techniques that make up lomilomi have been passed down from generation to generation by members of Hawaiian families and by Hawaiian shamans known as "Kahunas," who incorporate lomilomi massage as part of their healing rituals. Lomilomi was introduced to people outside the Hawaiian culture by Margaret Machado, who was born in Hawaii in 1916. Through her efforts, it has slowly infiltrated Western society.

Lomilomi as practiced in its traditional form includes various massage strokes and use of pressure on specific points in an effort to relieve acute or chronic tension. These points are like those used in **shiatsu** and **reflexology**, but the pressure is held for a shorter length of time. Unlike other massage forms, practitioners of lomilomi often use their forearms and elbows to massage and treat the points. After a lomilomi session, recipients take a steam bath and shower in order to eliminate the toxins that are released during the massage. Along with the physical relief provided by lomilomi, the technique also has a strong spiritual component, as practitioners emphasize that the special relationship between an individual and his or her god is of vital importance.

Lomilomi is used to treat various musculoskeletal conditions, and in Hawaii it is still used to relieve pain associated with childbearing. Like other massage methods, it helps increase circulation of blood and lymph, promotes elimination of toxins, and facilitates healing.

ALSO SEE massage

LooyenWork (LOO-en-werk) is a therapeutic practice that combines painless deep tissue work, environmental evaluation, and movement re-education in order to correct structural problems that have been brought about by emotional, physical, and psychological traumas. The creator of LooyenWork, Ted Looyen, firmly believes that correcting such problems should be painless and gentle. Using his background as a counselor, therapist, and bodybuilder as a foundation, he studied various therapies—including the **Feldenkrais Method**, **Aston patterning**, **rolfing**, and postural integration—and developed an approach that allows for the unique needs of each person.

A LooyenWork practitioner first completes a body assessment to identify the visible effects of the physical, emotional, and psychological traumas a person has experienced in the past. Then the client undergoes a series of treatments that are specially designed to address his or her particular problem. Treatments consist of gentle, yet deep, tissue massage that separates the tendons, lengthens chronically shortened muscles, and works out connective tissue adhesions.

LooyenWork is used to treat chronically tensed muscles, postural imbalances, back pain, and sports injuries.

Lysine (LI-seen) is an essential **amino acid**, which is required by the body to make collagen, a strengthening tissue that makes up much of the body. All the bone, cartilage, and connective tissue in your body contain lysine. Lysine also helps carry calcium molecules throughout the body and ensures that sufficient amounts of the mineral are absorbed by the intestines. This ability has led many nutritionists and physicians to recommend lysine supplements for women to help increase their calcium absorption and prevent osteoporosis. When taken with calcium, lysine supplements can increase calcium absorption by 20 percent. Up to 90 percent of people with herpes simplex who take lysine find that it halts the growth of the virus. Lysine is found in split peas, kidney beans, corn, and in small amounts in vegetables, fruits, grains, and nuts.

Macrobiotics (mak-ro-bi-AH-tiks), which literally means "great life," is both a way of eating and a lifestyle in which people are taught to live in harmony with themselves and with the world. Macrobiotics is not a therapy; according to macrobiotic philosophy, it is a way of life in which people's food choices help prevent disease and have a lasting, long-term effect on both their current and future health.

Macrobiotics is based on the Eastern concept of **yin and yang**, the two complementary opposite forces in the universe. All foods have either a yin or yang quality, and every person has unique needs for different yin or yang foods depending on physical, emotional, mental, and spiritual makeup and environment. Those who follow a macrobiotic lifestyle strive to maintain their bodies, minds, and spirits in a state of balance and harmony through the foods they eat.

Foods in a macrobiotic diet include unprocessed grains as the primary food, with certain vegetables (squash, carrots, onions, and cabbage) usually accompanying them. Seaweed is also a regular part of the diet; beans, nuts, seeds, and fruits also are eaten routinely but not always daily. Meat, poultry, and dairy products are not recommended, and some fish is allowed occasionally. Whenever possible, all foods should be organic and unprocessed.

Macrobiotics was introduced to the United States by Michio Kushi, who studied with the master of macrobiotics, George Ohsawa, in Japan. Kushi claims to have documented proof that a macrobiotic diet can eliminate diabetes and hypoglycemia. A macrobiotic lifestyle also can be used to treat heart disease, obesity, menstrual disorders, digestive conditions, food allergies, obesity, hypertension, and to accelerate the healing process following surgery or other trauma.

Magnetic Therapy is the application of special magnets to the body or exposure of the body to magnetic fields for healing purposes. Although ridiculed by some conventional physicians, magnetic therapy is used around the world by people seeking relief from various acute and chronic conditions.

Magnetic therapy is based on several basic facts. It is known that magnetic fields influence biological systems and that people are bioelectromagnetic systems that contain a magnetic field. Magnet therapy uses a natural magnetic field to help the body heal. Simply, the outer surface of all nerve cells has a positive charge while the inner portion of the cell has a negative charge. When people feel pain, what is happening is that the blood is supplying the positive-charged cell membrane with more potassium, which increases the positive charge. The amount of pain felt depends on the degree of pain stimulation. When a painful site is exposed to an alternative magnetic force, the magnetism helps return a normal charge to each cell.

The use of magnetic force dates back to at least the third century B.C. Lodestone, a natural magnet, was used to relieve muscle spasms and to treat gout. Magnets were used by the ancient Chinese, Indians, Hebrews, Egyptians, Arabs, and Persians. Magnetic therapy was introduced to

Western cultures by Franz Anton Mesmer, an Austrian physician, in the 1700s, although not much attention was given to it at the time.

Today, small magnetic patches applied like Band-Aids are used for relief of muscle pain and soreness. In some countries, such as Japan, magnetic devices are recognized as medical products. In the United States, the FDA has approved magnetic devices for bone healing and for magnetic resonance imagery (MRI) only.

Magnetic therapy may help acute conditions such as sprains, burns, cuts, broken bones, and strains. Some people with arthritis, degenerative joint disease, and diabetic ulcers also get relief from magnet therapy.
ALSO SEE energy therapies

Maitake (me-TAH-ke) *(Grifola frondosa)* is a medicinal mushroom that is also known as "hen in the woods" and "dancing mushroom." It is native to northeastern Japan and has been used by the Japanese for centuries for its ability to improve overall health and strengthen the body.

Maitake, like other medicinal mushrooms (see **reishi**, **shiitake**) is rich in polysaccharides, which are known to strengthen the immune system. Maitake contains the polysaccharide D-fraction, which may be helpful in treating cancer of the stomach, lung, and liver, as well as leukemia. According to studies published in the *Chemistry and Pharmacology Bulletin* (March 1992), maitake can kill the HIV virus and promote activity of T-cells in patients with HIV or AIDS. There are also reports that maitake can reduce blood pressure in people with mild to moderate hypertension.

Manual Lymph Drainage is a massage technique designed to improve the function of the lymphatic system. The lymph vessel system plays a major role in maintaining a healthy immune system, as it is responsible for transporting excess proteins, water, and wastes from the connective tissues to the bloodstream. Manual Lymph Drainage improves the flow of lymph and thus helps remove substances from the body tissues that can cause or contribute to disease.

Manual Lymph Drainage is the brainchild of two physical therapists working in France, Emil and Estrid Vodder, who, in 1932, began investigating ways to stimulate lymph and fluid movement. They developed some rhythmic manipulations, which they tested on people who had lymphedema, a condition characterized by tissue swelling (edema) triggered by blocked or damaged lymph vessels. After witnessing much success with their manipulative techniques, the Vodders established a systematic approach to treatment of the entire body and named it Manual Lymph Drainage.

Practitioners of Manual Lymph Drainage use slow, gentle, repetitive strokes to enhance the circulation of lymph, which naturally circulates more slowly than blood. Improved circulation of lymph is instrumental in healing many conditions. If connective tissue is damaged (e.g., burns, ulcers, inflammation, and so on), the lymph system carries the toxins and damaged cells away from the injured site. Use of Manual Lymph Drainage can facilitate recovery. Manual Lymph Drainage stimulates the nervous system and fluid movement in the connective tissues' cells and may have a beneficial effect on the immune system.

Marijuana *(Cannabis sativa L)* is a hardy plant that has been used for thousands of years to treat many different ailments, but perhaps is best known as an illegal recreational drug. Until 1937, it was legal in the United States for all purposes, medical as well as industrial and recreational. At that time, The Marijuana Tax Act of 1937 was passed, which established the federal prohibition of marijuana. Subsequently, The Controlled Substances Act of 1970 established five categories, or "schedules," into which all illicit and prescription drugs are categorized. Marijuana is a Schedule I substance, which means it is classified as having a high potential for abuse, no currently accepted medical use in treatment in the United States, and no accepted safety for use under medical supervision. Numerous studies since that time, however, have rediscovered many significant medicinal uses for marijuana.

Marijuana has therapeutic value in four general areas: relief from nausea and loss of appetite; reduction of intraocular (inside the eye) pressure; reduction of muscle spasms; and relief from mild to moderate chronic pain. For example, in patients with cancer, marijuana significantly reduces the nausea, vomiting, and loss of appetite caused by chemotherapy. People with AIDS get relief from the nausea, vomiting, and loss of appetite caused by the disease and by AIDS medications. The inner eye pressure and the accompanying pain that characterize glaucoma are both reduced with marijuana use. Some people with multiple sclerosis experience less muscle spasticity and tremor, improved gait, and better bladder control when using marijuana. Marijuana can also prevent epileptic seizures in some patients with epilepsy, and it can reduce chronic, debilitating pain. It is also reportedly helpful for people with migraine, arthritis, pruritus (severe itching), menstrual cramps, and depression.

Use of marijuana for medicinal purposes has been advocated by many respected institutions, including the National Academy of Sciences (1982), the California Medical Association (1993), the Federation of American Scientists (1994), the Australian Commonwealth Department of Human Services and Health (1994), the American Public Health Association (1995), the San Francisco Medical Society (1996), the California Academy of Family Physicians (1996), and several state nursing associations. As of early 1998, several states had passed state initiatives that approved medicinal use of marijuana but were facing legal challenges from the federal government.

Massage is hands-on manipulation of body tissues using stroking, rubbing, kneading, or other similar touch, or an appropriate instrument, for healing purposes. There are dozens of kinds of massage, which differ in ways such as intensity of treatment, types of strokes used, how it is applied (use of palms, fingers, elbows, knuckles, feet, knees, or massage tools), and area of the body treated. Generally, however, all forms of massage share several principles: they help improve circulation of blood and lymphatic fluid, stimulate the skin and nerve endings, promote release of endorphins, enhance overall body functioning and harmony, reduce stress, and release tension. These qualities make massage especially effective in treating circulation problems, heart disorders, high blood pressure, headache, insomnia, back and neck pain, depression, stress, and various muscular aches and pains associated with sports and physical exertion.

Cave drawings suggest that our ancestors practiced mas-

MASSAGE TECHNIQUES

Among Western methods of massage, the following techniques are commonly used with varying intensity, depending on the desired result.

Stroking (effleurage): slow, long, sweeping movements made with the hands close together and thumbs about one inch apart

Kneading (petrissage): fingers and thumbs roll and squeeze the flesh

Friction: firm, small, circular movements made with the fingers, heel of the hand, or thumb pads

Percussion (tapotement): quick, brisk chopping or slapping hand motions designed to stimulate rather than relax

Knuckling: small, circular movements with the knuckles, made while the hand is held in a loose fist

Pressuring: application of deep pressure on specific areas, using the thumbs' pads or forefingers

sage 15,000 years ago. Hippocrates, in the fourth century B.C., taught that "The physician must be experienced in many things, but most assuredly in rubbing." Many of the massage methods practiced in the United States are based on **Swedish massage**, which was brought to the States by Per Heinrick Ling after he visited China in the nineteenth century. **Deep tissue massage**, **Esalen massage**, neuro-muscular massage, and **sports massage** are some of the most popular variations of the Swedish method practiced in Western society, while **shiatsu**, based on the Chinese discipline of **acupuncture**, is also widely available. There are other therapies that incorporate some form of massage into their routines. These fall into the broader category known as **bodywork**, a generic term that refers to massage plus other forms of manipulation therapy. Examples include **Hellerwork**, **reflexology**, and **rolfing**.

Meditation is a way of focusing the mind into a state of relaxed and heightened consciousness and perception. It is practiced by people of many different cultures, religions, and philosophies; it can be a mystical experience or a prag-matic one, or anywhere in between. Meditation is not one but hundreds of different techniques whose purpose is to learn how to be without purpose. One of the most well-known forms of meditation is **transcendental meditation**; others include **relaxation response**, Siddha meditation, and Buddhist meditation. Regardless of the form it takes or who is practicing it, all meditation shares the common elements of stilling the mind, taking time out from the world, and focusing on the present.

A popular explanation of meditation is that it is about *being* and not about *doing*. When people just *are*, they ex-perience an internal calm that is both physical and mental. During meditation, the levels of natural relaxation hor-mones increase, heart rate and breathing rate decrease, and stress and tension melt away. Psychologically, people can "step back" from their thoughts, feelings, and habits. As the mind becomes uncluttered, stress and tension fade away and thinking becomes clearer and more focused.

There are two basic approaches to meditation: concentrative and **mindfulness**. In concentrative meditation, participants focus on something repetitive, such as breathing, an image, or a sound (such as a mantra) in order to still the mind and allow greater awareness. This form of meditation underwent scientific investigation in the 1970s by Drs. Herbert Benson and R. Keith Wallace, who revealed that concentrative meditation can decrease heart rate, breathing rate, and oxygen consumption.

Mindfulness involves allowing yourself to be aware of passing thoughts, feelings, and sensations without thinking about them or becoming involved in them. Some describe mindfulness meditation as a continuous act of letting go— not allowing yourself to become attached to any thought, emotion, or sensation.

Meditation helps people achieve feelings of peace, calm, and joy; reduce stress, tension, and negative feelings; ease hypertension, muscular aches and pains, chronic pain, breathing difficulties, circulation problems, headaches, and migraine; eliminate insomnia; and promote overall health and well-being. Though meditation is effective alone, it is often incorporated into other therapeutic practices, such as **acupressure**, **biofeedback**, **hypnotherapy**, **massage**, **music therapy**, **tai chi**, **visualization**, and **yoga**, among others.

Megavitamin Therapy see orthomolecular medicine

Melatonin (mel-a-TOE-nin) is a hormone produced naturally by the pineal gland, a pea-sized structure located deep within the brain. At about age forty, the body's production of melatonin decreases dramatically. Melatonin is also available as a nutritional supplement and is being marketed as a sleep aid, a sex aid, an immune system booster, and an anti-aging agent, among other claims.

Some of these claims appear to be true. Melatonin regulates the body's circadian rhythm (the sleep/awake cycle), influences the reproductive and cardiovascular systems, boosts the immune system, and enhances sleep. It is proven to help people fall asleep and to help those who wake up frequently to stay asleep. People who experience jet lag and those who work shifts or who have frequent schedule disruptions find that melatonin helps to restore the body's natural rhythms. It is also a very potent antioxidant.

Claims that melatonin enhances sexuality or can extend life appear to be wishful thinking. Russel J. Reiter, Ph.D., professor of neuroendocrinology at the University of Texas Health Sciences Center and author of more than 700 articles on melatonin, believes that although melatonin may help reduce symptoms of premenstrual syndrome, claims that it enhances sex have no scientific basis. Reports that melatonin can lengthen lifespan are based on studies done in rodents, which lived 20 percent longer when taking melatonin. However, melatonin can stimulate the immune system and protect the cardiovascular system, which does have an effect on lifespan.

Drugs and circumstances that can interfere with natural melatonin production and prompt the need for supplementation include lack of sunlight; ingestion of alpha- and beta-blockers and nonsteroidal anti-inflammatory drugs; exposure to electromagnetic fields, such as those associated with microwave ovens and electric blankets; and exposure to X rays and toxic chemicals.

Melatonin supplements are available in natural or synthetic form. The natural melatonin is extracted from the pineal glands of animals. It can vary greatly in potency and is much more expensive than synthetic melatonin, which is extracted from beans and is chemically identical to the melatonin produced by the body.

Mensendieck System is a movement therapy developed by a medical doctor for the purposes of improving the body's structural and functional integrity and eliminating any accompanying aches and pains. The system incorporates a program of "movement schemes" that are physically undemanding yet effective in invigorating, reshaping, and restructuring the body.

Bess Mensendieck (1861-1957) was one of the world's first female doctors when she graduated from the University of Zurich. During her work with paralyzed patients and the disabled elderly, she, along with her father, created a new system of functional body education. She tried to introduce her method to the United States in 1905, but the nude illustrations she used to demonstrate her work were censored. After establishing her method in Europe, she returned to the United States in the 1930s. Dr. Mensendieck's method was used by athletic departments, dancers, and actors, including Greta Garbo, Ingrid Bergman, and Fredric March.

The Mensendieck System consists of more than two hundred different exercises that focus on proper, graceful body movements in everyday activities. Mensendieck believed that the body is composed of a group of masses which need to be positioned correctly at rest and when in motion in order to avoid straining any of the muscle groups.

Teachers guide their students into various positions without demonstrating them but by using verbal and hand cues only. Mensendieck believes this process allows individuals to discover their own patterns of movement. The Mensendieck System reportedly is effective in people who have back pain, Parkinson's disease, sports-related muscle and joint injuries, fallen arches, and poor posture, as well as those recovering from surgery.

Meridians (muh-RIHD-ee-uhns) (also called organ meridians) are invisible pathways in the body that connect various **acupuncture** and **acupressure** points with the internal organs. Meridians serve as "highways" along which a person's vital energy, or **chi**, flows and circulates throughout the body. The Chinese believe chi flows from one meridian into another and completes one full cycle of the body per day.
ALSO SEE Chinese medicine; traditional Chinese medicine

MERIDIANS

Here are the 14 meridians, and their common abbreviations, referred to in acupuncture, acupressure, and other therapies involving chi.

Lu	Lung	LI	Large Intestine
Sp	Spleen	St	Stomach
H	Heart	SI	Small Intestine
K	Kidney	B	Bladder
TW	Triple Warmer	P	Pericardium
Lv	Liver	GB	Gall Bladder
CV	Conception Vessel	GV	Governing Vessel

Milk Thistle *(Silybum marianum)* is a thorny, weedlike plant that is used to make an extract called silymarin. This extract is rich in **flavonoids** that are especially beneficial for the liver; it boosts the regeneration of liver cells and increases the liver's ability to break down toxins and filter blood.

The ability of milk thistle to heal liver problems has been known since at least the first century A.D., when the Roman Pliny wrote that the fruit of the herb was "excellent for carrying off bile." Since then, milk thistle has been popular in Germany and other parts of Europe and is taken as a preventive measure against exposure to environmental and food toxins. It is available as a food supplement in the United States.

Mindfulness is a meditative state of awareness in which people are silent witnesses to their thoughts, emotions, actions, and the world around them. It is the art of becoming intensely aware of the present moment and accepting it as it is, without judgment.

Mindfulness is a Buddhist practice called *vipassana*, or insight meditation. Dr. Jon Kabat-Zinn, Ph.D., director of the University of Massachusetts Stress Reduction Clinic, author of *Full Catastrophe Living*, and an expert on mind-body medicine, notes that "the key to mindfulness is not so much *what* you focus on but . . . the quality of the awareness you bring to each moment." The practice of mindfulness can be formal or informal. Examples of formal mindful meditation include **yoga** and **tai chi**. Informal mindful meditation often takes the form of moments snatched during the day when people stop and consciously create a mindful experience. This can be as simple as taking several minutes to savor a grape: popping it into your mouth, rolling it around without puncturing it with your teeth, and enjoying how it feels in your mouth, then deliberately biting it and slowly chewing it, noting its sweetness and how the grape's skin gets between your teeth.

ALSO SEE meditation

Minerals are inorganic nutrients present in minute amounts in the body which are necessary for healthy functioning. In some cases, health-care practitioners suggest supplementation to address either mineral deficiencies or to treat specific symptoms and conditions.

Minerals are categorized as either essential minerals, essential trace minerals (also called trace elements), or non-essential minerals (see box). To qualify for the former category, the body must require more than 100 milligrams of the mineral per day; in the second category are all those of which the body requires less. Minerals in the latter category are toxic and have an imbalancing effect on the body. The two groups of essential minerals exist in relationship to one another and depend on proper diet, absorption ability, control of toxicities, and nutrient interactions to help maintain a healthy balance.

The government has established Recommended Daily Allowances (RDAs) for minerals. A recent study by the National Institutes of Health and other agencies finds that most people in the United States and other affluent countries do not reach even 75 percent of the RDAs for many trace minerals.

MINERALS

ESSENTIAL MINERALS	ESSENTIAL TRACE MINERALS	
calcium	chromium	molybdenum
chloride	copper	selenium
magnesium	cobalt	vanadium
phosphorus	fluorine	zinc
potassium	iodine	
sodium	iron	
sulfur	manganese	

In addition to taking mineral supplements to help meet RDAs, some supplemental minerals help relieve symptoms and treat disease. Calcium helps protect against osteoporosis and may help lower mild high blood pressure and reduce the risk of colorectal cancer. **Chromium** relieves symptoms of hypoglycemia, prevents some people from developing diabetes, and helps protect the heart and arteries. Copper helps regulate blood pressure, prevents heart rhythm problems, balances cholesterol levels, boosts the immune system, and protects against cancer. Magnesium protects against heart disease, reduces blood pressure, slows bone loss, prevents recurrent kidney stones, and strengthens muscles. Always take magnesium supplements with calcium. Manganese protects the bones and guards the body against heart disease and other degenerative diseases. Molybdenum helps prevent some cancers and guards against tooth decay. Supplementation with potassium can reduce blood pressure, protect against heart disease and stroke, reduce the risk of cancer, and prevent kidney problems. **Selenium** is an important **antioxidant**; it helps prevent certain cancers, improves circulation and rheumatoid arthritis symptoms, boosts the immune system, and improves mood.

Zinc enhances the immune system and appears to be especially helpful in warding off the common cold.

Mistletoe

(MIS-el-toe) (*Viscum album*, European species; *Phoradendron serotinum*, American species) is a parasitic shrub that grows in trees and which has a long history of use for treatment of conditions as diverse as epilepsy, menstrual cramps, typhoid fever, and arthritis. Ever since 1920, physicians in Europe have been using mistletoe to successfully extend the lives of cancer patients, but in the United States it is generally regarded as a poison by the Food and Drug Administration.

Mistletoe has had a see-saw history. Hippocrates advocated use of mistletoe for disorders of the spleen, but many other ancient physicians warned against internal use and recommended external use only. Physicians in seventeenth-century France and England used it to treat epilepsy and stroke and suggested wearing a sprig around the neck to "remedy witchcraft." In the nineteenth century, physicians were warned about the herb's toxic effects if taken in large amounts, namely vomiting, muscle spasms, convulsions, and coma.

Despite years of controversy about the opposite effects provided by European versus American mistletoe, analyses show that they have similar active components and thus similar effects: it slows the pulse, reduces blood pressure, and stimulates gastrointestinal and uterine contractions. To this list add the claims that it inhibits the growth of malignant cancer cells and destroys them. This finding was made by Austrian scientist Rudolf Steiner in the 1920s. Since then, mistletoe, available under the trademarked name Iscador, has been used by Europeans for cancer treatment. In the United States, health-care practitioners can use Iscador under the name Viscum Compositum.

Moxibustion

(moks-ih-BUS-chun) is the application of heat to specific points on the body, usually **acupoints**, in order to restore the normal flow of **chi** through the **merid-**

ians and thus promote healing. The skin is not burned during moxibustion.

Moxibustion can be done in several ways. One method involves placing small cones composed of dried leaves of the *Artemisia vulgaris* (called "moxa"), a species of chrysanthemum, directly on the skin. The tips of the cones are lit but extinguished when the recipient feels heat. Some acupuncturists burn moxa on the end of acupuncture needles to augment the effect. Another approach involves rolling moxa into sticks and holding the lit sticks close to the acupoints. If a large area needs to be treated, such as the lower back or kidneys, lit moxa can be placed into a special box and positioned over the affected spot. For very specific needs, moxa can be used with certain herbs. Moxa burned on a slice of ginger, for example, helps promote circulation, while a slice of garlic provides a strong antiseptic effect.

According to **Chinese medicine**, moxa has a pure yang nature and the ability to open up all twelve regular meridians. When burned over an acupoint, it can penetrate deep into the muscles, stop bleeding, regulate chi and blood flow, and eliminate coldness. Thus moxibustion is used to treat arthritis, neck and back pain and stiffness, fatigue, diarrhea, asthma, indigestion, and menstrual problems.
ALSO SEE acupuncture

Mushrooms (medicinal) include specific species of either wild or cultivated mushrooms consumed for their ability to boost the immune system. Mushrooms have been honored for millennia in China as tonics, for increasing resistance to stress and disease, and for extending longevity. Today they are popular around the globe, with worldwide sales exceeding one billion dollars, according to a 1993 report from the First International Conference on Mushroom Biology and Mushroom Products.

According to health expert Andrew Weil, M.D., author of *Spontaneous Healing* and *Natural Health, Natural Medicine*, most of the medicinal mushrooms grown in Japan and China have antiviral, antitumor, and immune-stimulating properties. Research indicates that polysaccharides—a type of sugar—are the components responsible for these healing properties. Increasing interest in the United States for medicinal mushrooms has spurred their availability and cultivation here. The most common medicinal mushrooms marketed in the United States are **shiitake** and **reishi**, although other varieties are available in the States and are grown here as well, including **maitake**, enokitake, and zhu ling.

Music Therapy is a treatment modality in which an individual who may have problems with emotional, physical, or psychological issues works along with a trained professional and uses music in systematic, creative ways to resolve those issues. Music therapy is effective in both children and adults and has proved particularly therapeutic in physically handicapped individuals. When they have the opportunity to express themselves creatively with music, they often discover previously unrealized talent and a new interest.

Music therapy allows for self-expression: people can choose from a variety of musical instruments, use their voices, or both, as ways to express their feelings, emotions, and energy in an acceptable way. Because music has structure—melody, tempo, rhythm, pitch, and so on—it requires people to pay attention to order and precision, which can be important, for example, in learning responsibility. A combination of guided **imagery**, **hypnotherapy**, or **biofeedback** and music is used by some therapists and physicians to help relieve chronic pain, lower blood pressure, regulate arrhythmias, ease migraine pain, and help a woman relax during childbirth. It is also useful in relieving asthma, insomnia, stress, grief, and depression.

Researchers are just beginning to understand how music heals. They know that music invokes complex chemical changes in the brain and affects the areas involved in thought processes, emotions, and even ''primitive'' functions, such as respiration and heartbeat. This connection leads some music therapists to emphasize that people who undergo music therapy need to be trained to combine the music with an awareness of the mind-body connection. In the area of pain relief, some experts believe that certain kinds of music cause the body to produce natural painkillers, or endorphins, the same chemicals that cause a natural "high" among many runners and people who meditate. The type of music people choose will depend on the desired goal and how their bodies respond to it. Although classical music is commonly used, jazz, blues, big band, and even rock and roll can be therapeutic.

Myofascial Release (mi-o-FASH-el) is a **bodywork** technique that releases constriction and tension residing in the soft connective tissue (or fascia) and thus helps restore balance to the body. Myofascial (*myo* means "muscle") Release was developed by John Barnes, a physical therapist who integrated his knowledge of **craniosacral therapy** with soft-tissue manipulation methods. The result is a therapeutic approach in which practitioners use their fingers, palms, forearms, and elbows to apply long, sustained pressure to stretch the fascia. As tension and constriction are released from the fascia, pain relief and improved movement and function are the result.

Myofascial Release reportedly is most effective in relieving chronic pain associated with muscle constriction, such as neck, back, and jaw pain; stress-related conditions; scoliosis; and recurring trauma, such as sports injuries.

Myotherapy (MI-oh-THER-uh-pee) (also called trigger point myotherapy) literally means "muscle therapy" and is the application of direct pressure to trigger points—painful areas where muscles have been irritated or injured and formed a knot—to relieve muscle pain. Myotherapists use their fingers, knuckles, and elbows to press for about seven seconds on irritated spots. This process is usually painful, but relief occurs once the knot is eliminated and the muscle is released.

According to myotherapists, trigger points begin to accumulate in the body even before birth and continue to do so throughout life. Myotherapists believe that trigger points lie dormant until something sets them off; for example, a fall, stress, an automobile accident, or even wearing tight shoes. Pain may then occur either at a trigger point or at a remote spot where the primary trigger point has "referred" the pain. These referral sites have been mapped, so myotherapists know which areas on the leg, for example, to treat for back pain. After pressure has been applied to the trigger points, stretching exercises are recommended to facilitate healing and to maintain flexibility.

Myotherapy is the offspring of a medical therapy called trigger point injection therapy, which was developed in the 1940s by Dr. Janet Travell to relieve the pain caused by trigger points. Rather than invade the body with a needle, Bonnie Prudden proposed that sustained, intense pressure applied to trigger points could achieve the same results. Myotherapy is used to treat chronic musculoskeletal pain.

N

Natrum Muriaticum is a powerful homeopathic remedy that is made from sodium chloride, or common salt. Rock or sea salts are usually used to prepare the remedies. Symptoms of thirst for cold liquids, headache that stems from eyestrain or the inability to focus the eyes, head pain with chills and fever relieved by sweating, dry mucous membranes that may include cold sores on the lips, and a watery or thick mucus discharge from the mucous membranes often follow an emotional episode such as loss, grief, rejection, or unrequited love. Natrum muriaticum benefits individuals who are emotionally sensitive, averse to fuss, independent, moody, and unpredictable. They often prefer to keep their feelings and emotions to themselves and prefer to be alone when ill. Symptoms are worse when individuals lie down, and better in open air.

ALSO SEE homeopathy

Natural Hygiene (also known as life science) is a health system that promotes the preservation and restoration of health by directing people to live in harmony with nature through a natural diet and wholesome lifestyle. One of the guiding principles of natural hygiene is the concept of "auto-intoxication": a buildup of toxins in the tissues, blood, and body fluids that occurs when poor lifestyle habits deplete the nerve energy reserves in the body. This self-poisoning, according to natural hygiene followers, is a primary cause of disease.

Some of the other guiding principles of natural hygiene include the following: the body is a self-supporting, self-healing, self-constructing organism that strives for and achieves health by continuously ridding itself of toxic wastes; disease is a natural process that restores the body and therefore should not be suppressed; drugs, herbs, and other medicines that suppress the eliminative processes should not be taken; refutation of the idea that microorganisms are the sole cause of disease; periodic fasting provides the ideal environment for the body to repair itself and eliminate toxic wastes; and adherence to a generally fruit-based diet.

The idea of natural hygiene originated in 1820 with the pioneering work of Drs. Isaac Jennings and Sylvester Graham, who laid the foundations of this health system. One hundred years later, Dr. Herbert M. Shelton established the fundamental principles of natural hygiene and wrote the classic book, *The Science and Fine Art of Food and Nutrition*. A more recent popular book by Harvey and Marilyn Diamond, *Fit for Life* (1985), introduced natural hygiene to a broad audience.

Naturopathy (nay-chuh-ROP-uh-thee) (also called nature cure) is a general term for a complete diagnostic and therapeutic system that encompasses a variety of therapeutic methods classified as "natural medicine." Typically these techniques include **acupuncture**, **herbal medicine**, **homeopathy**, **osteopathy**, **massage**, **hydrotherapy**, clinical nutrition, **Ayurvedic medicine**, and other natural modalities. The well-respected lecturer and author of natural health books, Michael Murray, N.D., of Bastyr University of Natural Health Sciences in Seattle, Washington, calls naturopathy "an amalgamation of all the healing arts of the past, but with modern scientific validation." It's a kind of blending of old world thinking with new world thinking.

As a concept, naturopathic medicine is millennia old, since the oldest medical techniques and remedies known to humans are natural. Introduction of a "structured" form of naturopathy in the United States is usually credited to Benedict Lust, who came to the U.S. from Germany in 1896. He secured his medical degree before founding the first school of naturopathic medicine. As the first graduating class entered the workforce in 1902, another naturopathic school began operating in Idaho under the guidance of Dr. James Foster. Interest in naturopathy grew rapidly, as did the number of practitioners and people seeking their services. As allopathic medicine and the pharmaceutical industry blossomed in the 1940s and 1950s, however, naturopathy lost popularity until interest in holistic healing emerged in the 1970s and 1980s.

A brief description of naturopathy's primary philosophies is as follows: the body has the power to heal itself, therefore all remedies and treatments should support self-healing rather than mask symptoms; symptoms are signals that the body is out of balance and are the way by which the body eliminates toxins and works to heal itself; all treatments should be as gentle and natural as possible; a person's physical, emotional, mental, social, and spiritual needs are all taken into account for diagnosis and treatment; good health is contingent on clean air, clean water, whole-

	Acupressure	Acupuncture	Aromatherapy	Apitherapy	Applied Kinesiology	Autogenic/Hypnosis	Bach Flower Remedies	Biofeedback	Chiropractic	Craniosacral Therapy	Feldenkrais	Guided Imagery	Herbal Medicine	e.g.: chamomile	echinacea	eyebright	feverfew	garlic
ACNE/SKIN DISORDERS								●	●						●		●	
ALLERGIES/ASTHMA	●	●	●	●			●						●	●		●		●
ANEMIA		●											●					
ARTHRITIS	●	●		●					●		●		●					
BACKACHE	●	●							●	●	●		●					
BURNS, BRUISES						●							●					
COMMON COLD			●										●			●		●
CONSTIPATION	●												●					
DEPRESSION		●	●	●	●	●		●	●				●					
DIGESTIVE PROBLEMS	●												●	●				
FATIGUE	●				●													
HEADACHE	●	●	●			●		●	●	●			●				●	
HERPES SIMPLEX			●	●									●	●	●			
HYPERTENSION	●	●						●				●	●					●
INSOMNIA			●					●				●	●	●				
MENSTRUAL PROBLEMS/PMS	●		●	●			●	●					●					
NAUSEA	●												●	●				
PAIN, CHRONIC		●				●		●	●	●	●		●					
TOOTH & GUM PROBLEMS	●	●											●	●				
URINARY DISORDERS									●				●	●				
YEAST INFECTIONS													●					

goldenseal	hawthorn	nettle	St. John's wort	skullcap	valerian	wild yam	Homeopathy: e.g. aconite	allium cepa	arnica	kali bichromicum	ignatia	nux vomica	phosphorus	sepia	Hydrotherapy	Massage	Meditation	Nutrition/Supplements	Osteopathy	Reflexology	Trager Method	Yoga
●							●								●			●		●		
	●						●											●				●
		●																●				
							●								●	●		●				●
					●		●		●		●										●	
●							●															
							●	●	●			●										
							●											●		●		●
		●														●	●					●
							●						●			●		●				
●				●	●		●							●	●	●	●	●			●	
	●						●															
				●			●									●		●				●
		●	●	●			●				●	●				●	●	●				●
						●	●									●				●		●
																				●	●	●
							●		●	●				●		●	●		●	●	
●							●									●		●				
	●						●									●						
●							●											●				

some food, exercise, and "right living" (adequate sleep, no tobacco, little or no alcohol, and so on); and naturopaths have the responsibility to educate their patients and encourage responsibility for self.

Naturopaths believe that illness seldom occurs if the body is kept clean internally, thus they often prescribe special diets, brief periods of fasting, or colon hydrotherapy to clear toxins from the gut and bowels. Another tenet of naturopathy is that the mind and body are inseparable and that emotional stress leads to physical ill health. These two concepts are the reason many ailing individuals are given a "prescription" to stay at a health spa, especially in European countries where naturopathy is practiced widely.

Overall, naturopathy provides nontoxic, noninvasive care to both prevent illness and treat acute and chronic problems that have not responded well to other complementary medical modalities. More than other medical traditions, it has a strong focus on and research-supported command of nutrition and supplementation.

Neem is the name of an herb extracted from a tree of the same name. A native of India, but also grown in Asia and in arid parts of Africa, the neem is an evergreen and a member of the mahogany family. Its umbrella-shaped leaves, as well as its bark, fruit, seeds, and oils are used for various medicinal purposes, as they have been for more than 4,500 years.

Neem has potent anti-inflammatory effects, which makes it useful for treating rheumatism, osteoarthritis, and other inflammatory conditions. One reason for its anti-inflammatory action seems to be associated with its ability to prevent the release of inflammation-producing chemicals in the body, such as prostaglandins. Neem also has been effective in alleviating fever in people with malaria and in fighting malaria parasites. Topical application of neem has successfully treated ringworm and scabies. Several studies suggest that neem may help reduce blood pressure and irregular heartbeat, and may help some people with diabetes reduce their insulin requirement.

Nettle (*Urtica dioica*), commonly called "stinging nettles" because of its many irritating hairs, is a widely used herb for conditions as diverse as gout, hay fever, and high blood pressure. It is a prolific plant that grows well in North America.

Nettle has been used since ancient times, when the juice was used to treat snakebites and scorpion stings. Early Europeans used it to treat tuberculosis, asthma, cough, scurvy, and nosebleeds. Among Native Americans, the women believed nettle tea eased childbirth, and mothers among the early settlers used it to increase their milk production. Today, researchers report that nettle may relieve the pain of gout and osteoarthritis, lower high blood pressure, help reduce fluid accumulation associated with congestive heart failure, relieve hay fever, and ease the bloating that occurs in premenstrual syndrome.

Neuro-Linguistic Programming (NLP) is the study of the way people receive and take in information, how they process it for themselves, and how they act on the results. In most basic terms, NLP consists of a set of models that allows people to study the relationship between a person and his or her experiences in the world, and how communication impacts and is influenced by subjective experiences.

The term "neuro-linguistic programming" comes from the disciplines that influenced its development: neurology, linguistics, and observable patterns (programs) of behavior. NLP was developed in the mid-1970s by John Grinder, a professor at the University of California, Santa Cruz; a graduate student, Richard Bandler; and several other colleagues. According to Judith DeLozier, one of the developers, NLP is "an accelerated learning strategy for detection and use of patterns in the world."

As a methodology, NLP provides practitioners with the

means to isolate skills, abilities, and behaviors from their usual contexts and allows them to study and transfer them to others. Given the subjective nature of NLP, it uses models of how things work rather than statistical formulae to help effect change in their clients. Many of the models used in NLP were created by observing people who did things very well. Practitioners can use models such as meta-model, metaprogram, sensory acuity, representational systems, and others.

NLP can be used to learn new behaviors and unlearn old or "bad" ones, and to help eliminate phobias. For example, an NLP practitioner who has a client who is afraid of snakes might use a model that answers the question: What can we learn about a person who has pet snakes and loves snakes so we can teach the phobic person to be comfortable around snakes? Once the NLP practitioner and client identify the factors that allow the pet owner to love his snake, the practitioner can use any number of techniques to help the client relearn his or her reaction to snakes.

Nutritional Therapies are nutrition-based approaches that focus on specific food and supplement intake in order to prevent medical problems and to maintain health. Many different foods and nutrients, in various combinations, can be considered as nutritional therapy. It is up to individuals and their health-care providers to choose the nutritional therapy approach that is best for them.

Certain foods and supplements—be they **herbs, amino acids, vitamins, minerals,** or enzymes—have demonstrated the ability to treat a particular medical condition, to help prevent development or progression of a disease, or to be key in maintaining optimal health. Any one or more of these foods or supplements can be included in an individual's nutritional therapy plan. Women who are pregnant or planning to become pregnant, for example, may want to take a **folic acid** supplement to help prevent birth defects. A dietary plan that consists of specific **antioxidants** is also an example of nutritional therapy. Other examples include

vegetarianism, **macrobiotics**, the **Hay diet**, **megavitamin therapy**, and eating plans that include low-fat, high-carbohydrate foods.

Nux Vomica *(Strychinos nux vomica)* is strychnine, a potent poison extracted from the seeds, leaves, and bark of the poison nut tree, which grows in China, Thailand, Australia, India, and Burma. Since at least the eleventh century, nux vomica has been used, in minute quantities, for various ailments.

Nux vomica gained some notoriety during the Middle Ages, when it was used as an antidote to the plague. Today, nux vomica is a staple among homeopaths, who prescribe it for indigestion, vomiting, diarrhea accompanied by abdominal cramps, nausea, constipation, hemorrhoids, and other digestive conditions that are prompted by suppressed emotions or excess intake of alcohol, caffeine, tobacco, drugs, or certain foods. Its effectiveness in relieving the symptoms of hangovers and other overindulgences has earned it distinction as the "party-lovers' remedy" among those who require its healing actions.

Women who experience early, heavy, or irregular menstruation or who feel faint before menstruation may benefit from nux vomica, as do those who have cramps, cystitis, frequent urination, labor pain, and morning sickness during pregnancy. Nux vomica has also proved effective in relieving colds characterized by a blocked nose at night and a runny nose during the day; retching coughs; flu noted by fever and shivering, aching muscles; and headache and migraine in which the head feels thick or as if a nail had been driven through the skull.

ALSO SEE homeopathy

O

Ortho-Bionomy (OR-tho bi-ON-uh-mee) is an educational movement therapy that teaches a person how to be more physically and energetically at ease with his or her body. *Ortho* means "correct use of," *bio* is "life," and *onomy* means "principles or laws that govern." Thus ortho-bionomy literally means "the correct use of the principles of life." It incorporates some of the principles of **osteopathy, craniosacral therapy, Aston patterning**, and the **Feldenkrais Method**. Ortho-bionomy has been nicknamed the "Homeopathy of Bodywork" because it involves augmenting a present condition in order to bring about healing and a cure.

Ortho-bionomy was developed by a British osteopath, Arthur Lincoln Pauls, who was also a practiced judo instructor. In judo, people follow other people's movements and energy in the direction they are moving and exaggerate that direction if possible. Yet Dr. Pauls' medical training, and his colleagues', did not adhere to this principle. Dr. Pauls then learned about the work of Lawrence Jones, D.O., an American who practiced and wrote about a technique called Spontaneous Release Through Positioning. Because this concept was closely associated with judo principles, Dr. Pauls studied Dr. Jones's work and expanded on his principles.

Ortho-bionomy is based on the concept that the human body knows how to heal itself. When people experience pain, the body positions itself in a way to try to relieve that pain. Ortho-bionomy exaggerates that position and thus shows the body, through gentle exaggeration, how to heal itself. The body usually responds, and the procedure is painless for the client and easy for the practitioner. The idea of exaggerated positioning is one of the principles of judo, **tai chi**, and other martial arts.

Treatment sessions consist of discovering optimal ways to perform routine movements and functions and replacing dysfunctional patterns with new, flexible ones. Ortho-bionomy can help people who have arthritis, muscle pain, rheumatism, sports injuries, postural problems, and emotional stress. It improves circulation and range of motion and increases relaxation.

Orthomolecular Medicine is a branch of nutrition science in which disease and illness are treated with very large doses of nutrients. Orthomolecular medicine is sometimes referred to as "megavitamin therapy," which is imprecise because the therapy consists of minerals, amino acids, enzymes, and other nutrients in addition to vitamins. The term (*ortho* is Greek for "right" or "correct") was first used by Nobel Prize winner Linus Pauling to describe an approach that stimulates healing by taking substances that are already found in the body.

Pauling believed disease could be eliminated if the body were given the "right" amount of molecules of nutrients through good nutrition. Doctors of orthomolecular nutrition recognize that although every person needs the same list of natural substances, such as **vitamins, minerals, amino acids**, enzymes, hormones, and trace elements, the exact amounts vary based on individual genetics, lifestyle, and environment. Disease results when the body has an excess or a deficiency of these natural substances and it cannot adequately restore damaged tissue. Treatment with nutrients allows the body to heal itself.

Orthomolecular medicine is controversial, and many conventional health care practitioners are hesitant to suggest it for their patients. Pioneers in orthomolecular medicine, however, including Linus Pauling and Jonathan Wright, M.D., have used megadoses of nutrients to successfully treat many ailments and diseases, including acne, allergies, anemia, common cold, chronic fatigue syndrome, hyperthyroidism, skin problems, heart disease, depression, infertility, viral infections, and others. Doctors of orthomolecular nutrition often recommend megadoses of nutrients for people whose nutrient levels are compromised because they smoke or drink large amounts of alcohol, or because they are chronically anxious or nervous. People whose diets contain much fat, preservatives, or caffeine also have an increased need for nutrients.

Osteopathy (os-tee-OP-uh-thee) is a medical discipline that combines manipulation of the musculoskeletal system with conventional allopathic medicine. One way in which osteopathic medicine differs from conventional medicine is that it uses a holistic approach and treats all aspects of a person—physical, emotional, spiritual, and mental—rather than the disease and symptoms alone. Thus osteopaths define health as being the optimal state of balance, or homeostasis, among all parts of the body.

Osteopathy was developed by Andrew Taylor Still, M.D. (1828-1917), who believed that how the body functions is determined by its structure. The word "osteopathy" reflects this belief: *osteo* refers to the skeletal system and *pathy* means dysfunction. The healthy flow of circulatory, nutritional, and neural forces is essential for good health; thus osteopathy emphasizes good nutrition, physical exercise, and healthy lifestyle habits. Osteopaths perform soft-tissue manipulation (e.g., various massage techniques) and soft-tissue mobilization (e.g., movement therapy, craniosacral manipulation, physical therapy) as needed for patients to regain or maintain optimum functioning of organs, muscles, tendons, ligaments, and other body structures.

Osteopathic physicians, or D.O.s (Doctors of Osteopathy) complete traditional medical training and then continue on to study manipulative procedures. They generally prescribe treatments and remedies that stimulate the body's natural ability to heal itself (e.g., herbal or homeopathic remedies, physical therapy, massage) and reach homeostasis. However, they can also prescribe drugs, perform surgery, and utilize other conventional medical techniques as needed.

Osteopathy is useful in the treatment of musculoskeletal problems, such as back pain, headache and migraine, arthritis, fibromyalgia, sports injuries, pregnancy discomfort, chronic pain, and most conditions that involve muscles or skeletal features. It also may speed up recovery from respiratory ailments, such as asthma, bronchitis, chronic obstructive lung disease, and sinusitis, as well as hasten recovery after surgical procedures.
ALSO SEE craniosacral therapy

Oxygen Therapy see hydrogen peroxide therapy; hyperbaric oxygenation therapy; ozone therapy

Ozone Therapy is the introduction of ozone (O_3) into the body for medicinal purposes. This therapeutic form is recognized in 16 countries and practiced mostly in Europe. It is available through approximately 300 physicians in North America.

Medical ozone is created when oxygen is electrically activated in an ozone generator. Once introduced into the body, ozone increases the oxygen level in the body, which is believed to help the immune system. Ozone therapy also promotes cellular respiration, which facilitates cell functioning.

Ozone can be delivered to the body in several ways. The most direct way is to mix ozone and oxygen into about one-half pint of the recipient's blood and administer the mixture intravenously. Other forms of administration include drinking ozonated water, encasing a limb or the entire body in a bag filled with ozone, breathing ozone bubbled through olive oil, or applying ozonated olive oil to the skin.

The first ozone generators were developed in Germany in 1857. By 1870, ozone was being used therapeutically to purify blood. More recently, German physicians have successfully used ozone to treat patients with AIDS (1979,

1980), while reports from Cuba claim ozone's effectiveness in treating glaucoma, conjunctivitis, and retinitis pigmentosa (1990). In 1992, the Russians revealed that ozone bubbled into brine is effective in the treatment of burn victims.

Physicians in the United States have treated dozens of diseases with ozone therapy, including candida, dermatitis, asthma, cancer, diabetes, and HIV-related conditions. The topical form is useful for cuts, scrapes, burns, rashes, insect bites, eczema, herpes, and other skin conditions.

ALSO SEE hydrogen peroxide therapy

Past Life Regression Therapy is a highly controversial form of psychological therapy that involves the use of hypnosis to help people remember their past lives. This technique, which originated in the 1960s, is used for individuals who, despite counseling or therapy, have a persistent irrational fear or who are "stuck" in their development. Some therapists believe the memories of past lives are true and find that helping clients access these memories can either eliminate the troublesome feelings or behaviors or at least provide their clients with a reason for why they feel or act the way they do. Critics of past life regression therapy say that people create past life scenarios or that the ideas are somehow planted in their minds. In either case, therapists can gain insight into how and what their clients are feeling by interpreting the information and behaviors clients reveal during hypnosis.

A pioneer in past life regression therapy, Brian Weiss, M.D., has worked with more than 1,400 patients and completed two books on the subject. He believes "When we understand reasons, patterns, and causes, we experience what many call Grace. The Grace of understanding allows us to transcend the traditional idea of karma, so that we don't have to reenact the same old dramas.'' Once people release themselves from repeating past mistakes, they can eliminate the pain and fear associated with them and move ahead with their lives.

Pau D'arco (paw de-AR-ko) *(Tabebuia heptaphylla)* is a tree that grows in Brazil, whose inner bark is used for its healing powers. In Argentina the same tree is called ''lapacho.'' According to the history records of the Calaway tribe, descendants of the Incas, pau d'arco is effective in the treatment of various cancers. Tea made from the bark reportedly ends pain in cancer patients and reduces or eliminates tumors. Herbalists use pau d'arco to treat ulcers, diabetes, rheumatism, osteomyelitis, leukemia, bronchitis, hemorrhage, gonorrhea, cystitis, gastritis, Parkinson's disease, arteriosclerosis, lupus, inflammation of the urinary tract, and anemia. Dr. James Duke, formerly of the National Institutes of Health, and Dr. Norman Farnsworth, of the University of Illinois, verify that pau d'arco contains cancer-fighting substances. The inner bark is the most potent part of the tree, although some companies harvest the outer bark.

Peppermint *(Mentha piperita)* is the most common and popular mint, with spearmint coming in a close second. Both peppermint and spearmint have similar healing properties, although peppermint is more potent and has more taste.

Until 1696, when botanist John Ray noted the differences between peppermint and spearmint, experts had not distinguished between the two species. Peppermint is a hybrid of spearmint and thus is a more recent arrival than spearmint. The mint mentioned as a stomach soother in the ancient papyruses of Egypt and throughout ancient Greece and Rome could have been of other species. Mint was prescribed as a digestive tonic and to treat colds, fever, and cough by Chinese and **Ayurvedic** physicians, as well as by English herbalists. Once John Ray noted that peppermint oil contains menthol and spearmint oil consists of the less potent carvone, herbalists considered peppermint to be the more effective remedy.

Peppermint is perhaps best known for its ability to soothe the stomach lining and to relieve flatulence, nausea, vomiting, diarrhea, and dysentery. Some herbalists recommend it for morning sickness. The essential oil of peppermint helps relieve nasal, chest, and sinus congestion when the vapors are inhaled. The oil is an effective antibacterial and also kills the virus that causes herpes simplex. This finding has led many herbalists to recommend it for the treatment of wounds, burns, and scalds, and for bronchitis. Peppermint can be used safely in infants to relieve colic and spasms and can be applied externally to relieve the pain of rheumatism, neuralgia, and headache.

Pet Therapy is the practice of bringing together companion animals and people for therapeutic reasons, as the presence of pets in people's lives has a healing effect on people as well as the pets. Many study results show that merely having a dog or cat or stroking it lowers blood pressure, reduces heart rate, and generally invokes a sense of calm among people of all ages.

Various animals are used in pet therapy programs, depending on the audience and the environment. Dogs and cats are the most popular, although birds, rabbits, guinea pigs, ferrets, and fish are other favorites. Many nursing homes and hospitals now have pet therapy days when animals are brought in to visit with residents and patients. Animals are also taken to correctional facilities, where a decline in destructive behaviors has been noted in many cases; and to facilities for the physically and mentally handicapped, where animals provide invaluable emotional and social healing.

Animals have the ability to evoke responses from otherwise nonresponsive people and provide individuals with something they can love and care for. Many experts believe the emotional bonds people form with animals help reduce or eliminate depression, stress, loneliness, and stress-related symptoms.

Pfrimmer Deep Muscle Therapy is a system that helps restore damaged muscles and soft tissues in the body. It was developed by Therese C. Pfrimmer, a massage therapist and physiotherapist from Canada, in the 1940s. Practitioners of this therapy are highly trained to use specific techniques of cross tissue movements as applied to the muscles. Therapists restore normal blood and lymphatic flow to all layers of muscle and thus promote the body's natural healing tendencies.

Phenylalanine (fen-il-AL-uh-neen) is an essential **amino acid** that plays a critical role in the body's metabolism. It is essential because the body cannot produce it and so needs to obtain it from the diet. **Bee pollen** is a good source of phenylalanine.

Phenylalanine is the "source material" for production of specific neurotransmitters called catecholamines, of which the best known is adrenaline. Maintaining an adequate level of phenylalanine in the body is necessary for mental alertness, positive mood, and a sufficient level of adrenaline, which helps people cope with stress. Phenylalanine can be used to treat depression, especially that associated with premenstrual syndrome and menopause. When combined with **tyrosine**, phenylalanine can stimulate the thyroid gland and boost the metabolism rate, which can help in weight loss. Phenylalanine also prompts the intestines to produce a hormone called cholecystokinin, which sends a message to the brain that you are full and thus curbs appetite.

Phosphatidylserine (fos-fuh-TID-el-SER-een) is a naturally occurring phospholipid nutrient found in humans. Though it has a role in the functioning of nearly all cells in the body, it is most prevalent in the brain, where it performs many significant functions among the nerve cells, including the conduction of nerve impulses and the accumulation, storage, and release of neurotransmitters.

The high concentrations of phosphatidylserine in the brain cells led scientists to investigate its possible association with cognitive function. Recent studies suggest that dietary supplementation of phosphatidylserine may support cognitive functioning and slow mental decline as people age. The nutrient appears to achieve this in an indirect manner. Membranes make up the primary work surfaces of cells, and nerve cells depend on membranes to perform specific processes. Phosphatidylserine is a membrane-active nutrient, and as such it helps stimulate and regulate many of the proteins that are involved in these processes.

Phosphorus (FOS-for-us) is an essential element in the functioning of human cells. In **homeopathy**, it is a remedy derived from bone ash that is often used to treat a variety of conditions that result from a dysfunction of tissue or cell metabolism. It is often prescribed as a constitutional remedy for young people who are growing rapidly and who suffer with apprehension over taking exams. Symptoms may include flushes of heat, rising upward from the chest, in people who are susceptible to palpitations and congestion; hemorrhaging; anemia; extreme thirst for ice-cold fluids; extreme hunger, often accompanied by or preceding a headache; hoarseness that is worse in the evening; constriction and oppression in the chest; and congestive, throbbing headache that is worse for heat, lying down, and motion and better for cold and rest. A phosphorus personality is characterized by individuals who display intelligent cooperation, a need for affection and the ability to return it, and who are easily exhausted.

Pilates Method (pie-LAY-tez) is a series of movement exercises designed to strengthen and stretch muscles, release tension in the body, and open up joints. It was developed by Joseph Pilates (1880-1967), who believed that corrective exercise should begin with education and conditioning of the entire body.

Pilates noted that everyday activities can strengthen some muscle groups but leave many others weak and undeveloped. The Pilates Method was developed to provide a balance of strength and function among the muscles. It consists of more than 500 unique controlled movements performed on a series of five pieces of exercise equipment. The movements are done with controlled breathing and are designed to emphasize alignment and facilitate muscle balance as they focus on strengthening the lower back and abdomen, which are the power center of all movement. If the power center is strong, the rest of the body can move freely.

The benefits of the Pilates Method include increased muscle strength without adding bulk, increased flexibility, improved posture, and prevention of muscle and soft tissue damage. It is used by dancers and by professional and Olympic athletes and is popular in fitness centers. The method is accessible to everyone, including the elderly, pregnant women, and the physically challenged.

Polarity Therapy (po-LAR-ih-tee) is an integrated healing technique that restores energy balance to the body. It is based primarily on **Ayurvedic** philosophy, which states that a vital life force exists in and surrounds all living things. In polarity therapy, this energy force is recognized as an electromagnetic energy pattern. The vital life force flows through the body in bipolar currents, with the positive charge at the top of the head and the negative charge at the feet. When the energy force is hindered or disrupted, illness and disease occur. Polarity therapists use their hands (right hand is positive, left, negative) to establish a connection between themselves and their client and thus reestablish and rebalance the energy flow.

Polarity therapy was developed by Dr. Randolph Stone (1890-1981), a Viennese-born osteopath, chiropractor, and naturopath who extensively studied various healing practices from around the world before he developed polarity therapy. The therapy consists of four phases: gentle hands-on bodywork to facilitate energy flow and harmony; counseling on nutrition and diet; psychological counseling; and polarity yoga exercises. The connection is made using gentle direct pressure, shaking movements, or rocking motions. After the bodywork portion of the treatment, therapists typically offer dietary and nutritional counseling, which is basically vegetarian, as well as teach yoga exercises to augment the bodywork treatment and to stretch and balance the body. Emotional support that promotes positive thinking and provides encouragement is also offered by many polarity therapy practitioners.

Polarity therapy can be used to help prevent illness and facilitate healing. It has been successful in relieving pain associated with headache, muscle tension, low back pain, and digestive disorders as well as providing comfort for people with stress-related emotional problems.

Prayer, an invocation to God or other Higher Power for healing, good health, and other requests, has been called the universal remedy. Prayer is people's link between themselves and their God and can help the body and mind heal, if people truly believe, or have faith, that it will.

There seems to be little doubt that prayer can heal, regardless of the technique or style used. Exactly how it works is not known. Some people regard it as a visualization technique. Prayer helps put the mind at peace, and when there is less mental stress, the body is better able to heal itself. Prayer should not be regarded as a substitute for medical treatment, however, although some people have claimed miracle cures from cancer and other life-threatening conditions with the use of prayer.

People who practice prayer report that it is very calming and meditative. Besides the relaxing effects enjoyed by individuals engaged in personal prayer, intercessory prayer—when one person or more prays for other people—has been found to be effective.

The power of prayer has caught the attention of the Office of Alternative Medicine at the National Institutes of Health in Washington, D.C., the Mind Science Foundation, and other investigative organizations. Research into the effectiveness of prayer is ongoing and supported by many in the medical arena.

Primal Scream Therapy is a method that helps people confront and deal with unresolved, unfulfilled issues that formed during the time they were infants up to and including their childhoods. It is based on the concept that children often feel responsible when bad things happen to them; for example, their parents get divorced, a parent or sibling dies, or the child is sexually or emotionally abused. When they take the burden of guilt upon themselves, they label themselves as wrong, unworthy of love, and guilty. Carrying this burden into adulthood often results in people who have problems with relationships, who lack self-esteem and self-confidence, and who may unconsciously pass along these dysfunctional behaviors and feelings to their children.

Primal scream therapy was developed in the late 1960s by Arthur Janov, an American psychiatrist who studied the teachings of Sigmund Freud and Wilhelm Reich. It focuses on the cause of the types of unresolved emotional issues mentioned above and allows adults to release the pain and anguish associated with them by providing them with a safe environment in which to express their anger, fear, and other hurt feelings. Such an environment often consists of a darkened room, perhaps padded and sound-proofed as well. Despite its name, not all patients scream during therapy sessions. Most people who do primal scream therapy go for nine to twenty-four months of both group and individual sessions.

Propolis (PRO-po-lis) is a sticky substance that bees collect from the buds of trees. Bees use propolis to patch cracks and holes in the hive to protect against invasion by microorganisms. This practice makes beehives the most hygienic structures in the natural world.

Propolis has been dubbed the earliest known antibiotic, as Aristotle recommended it to treat bruises and sprains. Egyptian priests used propolis to disinfect and treat wounds, and the Incas used it to treat flu. Injured soldiers during the Boer War in the 1890s had their wounds disinfected with propolis. In the 1960s, two researchers at the Center of Biotic Research, Drs. Lavie and Vosmjak, described propolis as a nontoxic antibacteriologic agent that cannot be reproduced in a laboratory. Today, propolis is recognized for its antibiotic abilities and for being effective against inflammation of the mouth and throat, tonsillitis, cold, flu, and cough, and as an immune system stimulant. It also can be applied to bruises and blemishes to facilitate healing.

Propolis is rich in the B vitamins, vitamins C and E, beta-carotene, and twenty-one **amino acids**. It also contains 124 bioflavonoids and trace **minerals**. Supplements are available in tablets and extracts. For best results, take propolis with supplements of vitamin C and zinc. Among many Europeans and Russians, propolis is believed to be the optimal preventive medicine.

ALSO SEE apitherapy

Psychic or Spiritual Healing is based on the belief that the "laying on of hands" by healers transfers healing energy to ailing recipients. Some healers say their ability comes to them from God or a higher being; others say they are empowered by angels or spirits. Those who practice psychic or spiritual healing come from a wide diversity of ethnic backgrounds, religious beliefs, and philosophical followings.

"Laying on of hands" is a slight misnomer, as not all psychic or spiritual healers physically touch their clients; some healers work only in the energy field that surrounds the body. Psychic healing can take many forms and sometimes incorporates the use of music, crystals, sound, massage, or color to augment the healing experience.

Many medical professionals are skeptical of the claimed benefits of psychic healing, which are many: both healers and their satisfied clients claim psychic healing can alleviate or cure any physical, mental, or emotional problem. Much of the success of healing seems to hinge on the relationship between the healer and the client.

Psychic healers have been practicing for millennia and exist in most cultures. Acceptance of their skills varies greatly. While British physicians welcome psychic healers into their hospitals and clinics, for example, healers are banned in some states and are imprisoned in Germany.

Psyllium (SIL-ee-um), the seeds of the fleawort plant, is a natural laxative that is rich in soluble fiber. It is also popular as a cholesterol-lowering agent.

Psyllium softens stools naturally and makes it easier for the colon to pass and eliminate them. Psyllium seeds can be bought whole or ground in health food stores, or they are available as the primary ingredient in many over-the-counter laxatives.

For people with high cholesterol levels, many medical experts recommend taking psyllium daily to bring those levels down. The addition of psyllium to the diet can also reduce the risk of cancer of the colon or rectum.

Pulsatilla (pul-suh-TEE-ah) *(Pulsatilla nigricans)* is a homeopathic remedy prepared from the windflower plant, also known as the field anemone or pasque flower. It is a native of Europe. Generally, the remedy is most effective in people who are cheerful, gentle, and nervous, and who are fair-skinned, fair-haired, and plump. Pulsatilla is a popular remedy for children and adolescents. Some of the most common symptoms that respond to pulsatilla include digestive problems that are usually worse in the morning; thick, yellow-green discharge from the nose; one-sided headache, chills, or sweating; itching eyelids or sties; nosebleeds; flushed face; thirstlessness, even in the presence of a fever; and coated tongue and bad taste in the mouth. Patients are much worse for heat and rich, fatty foods; they are better for cool, open air and slow, gentle movements.

Pulsatilla is commonly used to treat cramps that accompany irregular menstrual flow and for cramps that are experienced in the lower back or kidney area and feel as though they are cutting and tearing. For women with morning sickness, pulsatilla works best in those who are cheerful and who feel warm, especially at night. During the third to sixth month of pregnancy, pulsatilla can help relieve heartburn, shortness of breath, and indigestion. Among women who become weepy and tearful premenstrually and who crave sweets, pulsatilla can offer relief.

ALSO SEE homeopathy

Pycnogenol (pick-NAH-geh-nol) is the patented name of a natural compound that is a potent **antioxidant** and a rich source of special **flavonoids** known as proanthocyanidins and many other beneficial components. Pycnogenol is derived from the bark of the French maritime pine tree and has been the subject of extensive testing, which shows it to be effective in the treatment and prevention of many medical conditions.

As an antioxidant, pycnogenol has been shown to be fifty times more effective than vitamin E and twenty times more effective than vitamin C. Because it can readily pass into the brain, it is able to protect the cells and blood vessels in the brain from free-radical damage and thus help memory and reduce senility. There are also some indications that pycnogenol helps reduce attention deficit disorder. Pycnogenol is a popular supplement for the prevention of varicose veins, poor circulation, and fragile capillaries. As an antiinflammatory it is often taken to treat arthritis. Pycnogenol also stabilizes collagen, an essential protein in maintaining the health of the skin, joints, and blood vessels. Its ability to revitalize collagen makes pycnogenol popular among people who want to maintain a youthful complexion.

Q

Qigong (che-kung) is an ancient Chinese tradition that combines regulation of posture, mind, and breath as a way to promote health, well-being, and longevity, and to cure ailments and disease. Some who practice qigong also incorporate self-massage and movement of the arms and legs with the torso.

The word "qigong" is composed of *qi,* "vital energy" and *gong,* "work" or "exercise"; thus qigong means "exercise with your vital energy." Qigong is practiced in many forms, but generally it is divided into five schools—**Taoist,** Buddhist, medical, martial art, and Confucian—of which the first two are the most popular. Both of· these methods concentrate on movements that help bring the body into balance and clear the mind. Taoist involves gentle, steady movements that move from soft to hard, while Buddhist uses dynamic motions that move from hard to soft. Medical qigong consists of theory only and involves acupuncture. Martial arts includes specialized training, and Confucian is rarely practiced today.

When people practice qigong, there are four key areas on which they need to concentrate: the dantien, or "center," which is the area within every person that stores qi energy; the mind, as they strive to keep it clear and calm and try to become one with the universe; breathing, which should be in synch with their movements; and the body, as they focus on their movements and posture.

Qigong has proved useful in the treatment of conditions such as hypertension, asthma, arthritis, neurasthenia, insomnia, fatigue, constipation, poor circulation, headache, and myalgic encephalomyelitis. It also is very effective as a stress reducer, and many athletes use it to improve performance.

R

Radionics (ray-dee-OH-niks) is a psychic method of making medical analyses at a distance using special instruments that reportedly can detect a person's energy state and vibrations. This form of healing actually has two steps: clients complete a detailed questionnaire and practitioners also ask for a "witness"—a drop of blood or a lock of hair that can be assessed and used to arrive at a diagnosis or recommended treatment.

Radionics practitioners use both their natural sensitivity and scientific knowledge to identify imbalances in people's energy fields. They believe that the answers to diagnostic and treatment questions come to them from the client's unconscious mind and therefore may be "felt" intuitively or by observing the swing of a **dowsing** pendulum. Practitioners then determine the type of treatment needed, whether it be conventional, radionic healing, complementary, or a combination. Radionic treatment takes two forms: healing energies can be "broadcast" psychically (explained below) or transferred to sterile sugar tablets and taken orally by the client. This latter method is similar to a homeopathic approach.

Radionics was developed by Albert Abrams, an American neurologist who created a "black box," which, without the help of any electronic parts, he claimed could detect vibrations from a witness placed in the box and then transmit, or broadcast, healing radiations to the person from

whom the witness came. Many consider this to be a form of **psychic healing**. Conditions radionics may treat include allergies, asthma, eczema, arthritis, rheumatism, chronic pain, postsurgical pain, headache, migraine, and sleep disorders. Radionics reportedly can even reduce the severity or slow the progression of inherited conditions.
ALSO SEE energy therapies

Rebirthing Therapy is a process that allows people to access suppressed feelings associated with the personal birth experience and to release them in a safe environment so healing can occur. Rebirthing therapy helps restore physical, emotional, and mental balance to individuals who have unresolved emotional blocks and trauma.

The technique involves trained facilitators, or rebirthers, who guide clients through conscious breathing exercises that allow them to relive birth and face the fears, anxieties, and other repressed feelings associated with the event. The release of this repressed trauma is believed to restore physical, emotional, mental, and spiritual balance to people who have unresolved emotional issues.

Reflexology (ree-flek-SOL-uh-jee) (also known as zone therapy) is a manipulation technique in which various specific points—most often on the feet but occasionally on the hands as well—are pressed, massaged, and/or stroked in order to improve circulation, relieve stress and tension, and reduce pain. Reflexology is based on the concept that the soles of the feet are a ''map'' of the entire body: specific points called reflex zones are associated with organs, glands, and other body parts. When these reflex zones are pressed or massaged, the areas of the body that correspond to those zones are affected. Thus a reflexology treatment to the area of the foot associated with the head may bring headache pain relief, while stimulation of the large colon zones may ease constipation.

Reflexology is based on several ancient healing techniques and is similar in principle to acupressure: it stimulates the body's energy flow to allow the body to heal itself naturally. Archaeological evidence suggests that reflexology was practiced in ancient Egypt and Greece, and reflexologists believe the natives of North and South America used it as a form of healing. Reflexology evolved into its own form in the early 1900s with the work of two medical doctors: William H. Fitzgerald and Edwin Bowers. Physiotherapist Eunice Ingham elaborated on their work and created a map of the body as represented on the soles of the feet. Several variations of reflexology have emerged, including Morrel reflexology and the Vacuflex system.

Reflexology can be used as preventive therapy and to treat a wide variety of existing conditions. It seems to be most effective in the treatment of digestive problems, fatigue, aches and pains, inflammatory skin conditions, problems associated with pregnancy, stress and stress-related disorders, and menstrual irregularities.

Reichian Therapy (RIK-ee-uhn) is considered to be the great-grandfather of many modern **bodywork** therapies. Reichian therapists use a combination of physical movements, postural adjustments, and bodywork manipulations to release tension and repressed emotions.

Dr. Wilhelm Reich, a theoretician who was part of Freud's close circle of friends, believed that increased awareness of the body and a release of emotions were necessary for healing. Reich was, according to Joseph Heller (see **Hellerwork**), "the first Westerner to concentrate attention on the relationship between body tensions and rigidity, and psychological limitations to a person's well-being." During one-on-one sessions, Reich would assess a client for areas of the body that harbored blocked energy. Such areas are "armor" that the body creates to cope with a physical or emotional injury. To dissolve these blocks, Reich used both physical manipulation and psychoanalysis.

Reich died in 1957, and renewed interest in his work developed in the 1970s. From that interest has emerged several branches of neo-Reichian therapy, including **bio-energetics** and radix.

Reiki (RAY-kee), a Japanese word that literally means "universal life energy," is a healing technique that involves the laying on of hands and use of highly focused visualization as a way to restore a person's balance on all levels of existence: physical, spiritual, emotional, and mental.

Reiki as it is practiced today is based on ancient Tibetan Buddhist concepts that are approximately 10,000 years old. The core of this belief system is that each person possesses a universal life force that is accessible to him or her. Reiki practitioners say most people, however, have blocked their ability to tap into this energy. The role of reiki practitioners is to revitalize and unblock the energy flow. In order to do this, practitioners must first do attunements, initiations that open up and clear the channel through which the universal life force will flow via the practitioner to the client, or "receiver." Practitioners tap into a receiver's energy by gently placing their hands on various areas of the body that correspond to the **chakras**, the major organs, and the glands. Practitioners then channel reiki energy to the receiver and help restore harmony and balance.

Reiki was introduced to the modern world by Dr. Mikao Usui, a theology professor in Kyoto, Japan, in the mid-1800s. Dr. Usui set out to discover the secret of healing. In doing so he studied various healing techniques from many cultures. After studying some ancient Sanskrit Buddhist manuscripts given to him by a Zen Buddhist monk and meditating on the texts for many days, he had a vision that convinced him he had found the answer. Since then, the Reiki tradition has been passed down through highly trained individuals called Reiki Masters to patients and students. Reiki was brought to the United States in the 1940s by a Japanese-American woman named Hawayo Takata, who followed Usui's teachings. Today there are several variations of Reiki being practiced.

No one is certain how Reiki works, but its proponents believe it affects the chakras, which in turn stimulate the body's endocrine system. According to Reiki practitioners, disease results when emotional and mental states are out of balance. Reiki can both help prevent disease by maintaining balance in the body and hasten healing by restoring balance. Reiki is used to reduce stress and restore energy; treat acute and chronic physical ailments by promoting balance and well-being; heal emotional problems; and enhance personal growth.

Reishi (REE-shee) (*Ganoderma lucidum*; also known as ling zhi) is a medicinal **mushroom** that has been used by the Chinese and Japanese for thousands of years as a tonic to promote long life and overall good health. The late Hiroshi Hikino, the world's authority on Oriental medicinal plants, called reishi one of ''the most important elixirs in the Orient.''

In the sixteenth-century Chinese pharmacopeia *Pen T'sao Kang Mu*, which contains hundreds of natural medicines the Chinese have used for thousands of years, it is written that reishi ''positively affects the life energy, or qi of the heart, repairing the chest area and benefiting those with a knotted and tight chest. . . . Taken over a long period of time, agility of the body will not cease, and the years are lengthened to those of the Immortal Fairies.'' Today in China, reishi is used to fight the effects of stress, stimulate the liver, cleanse the blood, lower or raise blood pressure, beautify the skin, and fight hair loss. Injections of the spores are used to treat lupus.

Reishi's long history of success in Asia recently sparked interest in the West, where it is now being used to treat allergies, chronic fatigue syndrome, diabetes, liver disease, and immune-compromised conditions. It is also being used to treat neuromuscular conditions, such as myasthenia gravis and muscular dystrophy, but with varying degrees of success. Its medicinal value is believed to be at least partly related to the fact that it contains the immune system boosters polysaccharides, and that it is a potent **antioxidant**.

As recently as the 1970s, reishi was rare and difficult to cultivate. Scientists have now developed the delicate artificial growing conditions needed to grow the reishi mushroom.

ALSO SEE shiitake

Relaxation Response is a phrase that describes a natural relaxed state of mind and body that is characterized by various physiological changes. This response was discovered by Herbert Benson, M.D., of Harvard Medical School, and his colleagues, in 1974. At the time, they were conducting studies of the effects of meditation on breathing rate, brain wave patterns, and other physical factors and discovered that the body has its own stress-reducing mechanisms. The phrase "relaxation response" was coined by Dr. Benson to describe the body's reaction to stress.

How people react to stress is determined largely by the autonomic nervous system. This system is composed of the sympathetic nervous system and the parasympathetic nervous system. It's the latter system that helps the body relax by lowering heart rate and blood pressure and relieving muscle tension.

The relaxation response can be induced in many ways, including **meditation**, **visualization**, **prayer**, **breathing therapy**, **yoga**, **sound** and **music therapies**, **tai chi**, guided **imagery**, and other similar techniques. Any one or more of these approaches can allow people to enter a state of peace and calm, which in turn relieves tension held in the muscles and cells throughout the body. As tension is relieved, relaxation takes its place. The relaxation response is a natural complement to these and other natural therapies as well as conventional treatments.

In addition to physical changes, the relaxation response also causes the following changes: reduced respiratory rate, reduced oxygen consumption, reduced blood flow to skeletal muscles, and reduced perspiration. Regular practice can help relieve and prevent headache, back and neck pain, depression, chronic muscle tension, insomnia, hypertension, and other stress-related conditions.

Rolfing (also called structural integration) is a technique that involves manipulation of the body's myofascial system (the muscles [myo] and connective tissues [fascia]) in order to improve movement, balance, and support among the various parts of the body. It is performed by individuals, known as "rolfers," who have been trained in the technique.

Ida P. Rolf, Ph.D. (1897-1979), a biochemist who developed this bodywork technique in the 1960s, believed that the shape of the body reflects how well it functions and is balanced in relation to gravity. Rolfers correct the body's structure by stretching shortened connective tissues and returning them to their normal length and flexibility. Rolfing sessions involve repositioning various body segments, including lining the legs up with the feet, centering the pelvis over the legs, positioning the torso upon the pelvis, and balancing the head and neck evenly on the upper torso. As the body is placed into balance, overall health improves: connective tissues become healthier and more toned, bodily fluids flow more easily, the nervous system functions more smoothly, waste removal is more efficient, and breathing improves.

Rolfing also has an emotional side. Dr. Rolf consulted with Frederick S. Perls, the founder of **Gestalt therapy**, from whom she recognized the mind-body connection, or the link between emotions and muscle tone and function. Many people, she said, hold muscular tension in the body for years, often since childhood, as part of a learned behavior. For example, you may have been frightened by a German shepherd when you were five years old and you still unconsciously cringe whenever you see one. During rolfing sessions, the tension associated with this behavior can be released, and the emotional issue along with it. Thus emotional benefits can include an increased sense of well-being and relaxation. A balanced body operates to its maximum potential and utilizes energy well.

A typical rolfing course of therapy consists of 10 sequential sessions, each lasting sixty to ninety minutes, and can be painful. Despite the pain, people who have been "rolfed" report relief from chronic headache, postural problems, and chronic body aches and pains. Many of them return for follow-up treatments six months to two years later to address specific problem areas. Several scientific research studies have also shown rolfing to be effective in improving muscular efficiency, reducing anxiety, and decreasing pelvic tilt.

ALSO SEE Hellerwork

Rosen Method (ROE-zen) is a form of gentle bodywork that incorporates verbal communication and seeks to relieve muscular pain, reduce the effects of stress, and increase vitality and health. The primary role of a Rosen Method practitioner is to create an environment in which people can become aware of the connection between body, mind, and spirit and, in this awareness, come to know themselves in a more profound way.

This healing technique was developed by Marion Rosen (b. 1914), who, as a physical therapist, became interested in the fact that as her clients' muscle tensions resolved, they would reveal their inner feelings and emotions to her. Rosen believed that this constituted a release of pain by her clients and was an acknowledgment of an effort to make positive change. Thus Rosen practitioners gently touch and/ or use words to help their clients relax and release chronic muscle tension.

Marion Rosen founded the Rosen Method training program in 1972. Those trained in this method strive to prevent illness and disease by showing people how to become more aware of unconscious chronic stress and tension and the steps to eliminate them. Benefits of the Rosen Method include: reduction or elimination of muscle tension and pain, headache, irritability, and fatigue.

Royal Jelly is a thick, milky white substance that is secreted from the pharyngeal glands of bees, specifically the worker bees. All bees eat this nutritious and highly concentrated food during their first three days of life, but then switch to pollen after that time. Future queen bees, however, continue to eat royal jelly for the rest of their lives. Many bee experts believe this diet of royal jelly is responsible for the very long life of queen bees (four to five years) compared with the short lives (40 days) of other bees. Some health enthusiasts believe royal jelly may also help increase the longevity of human lives as well.

Among Chinese herbalists, royal jelly is recommended for liver disease, rheumatoid arthritis, anemia, gastric ulcer, physical weakness, and phlebitis. Western herbalists and other natural health practitioners often use it to nourish the skin, help prevent wrinkles, and improve sexual performance, and to treat depression, fatigue, and menopause. It also has some antibacterial benefits and can help stimulate the adrenal glands, which in turn increases metabolism and enhances energy.

Extensive testing of royal jelly has revealed that it is a rich source of complete protein (it contains all the essential **amino acids**), as well as natural sugars, biotin, and minerals. It is also the richest natural source of vitamins B5 and B6, which are important in the metabolism of carbohydrates and fats. Royal jelly is also a significant source of acetylcholine. This substance regulates the nerve impulses between the nerve fibers and is deficient in people with Alzheimer's disease. Some researchers claim that supplements of royal jelly result in improved physical and mental stamina in patients with Alzheimer's.
ALSO SEE apitherapy

Rubenfeld Synergy (ROO-ben-feld) is a combination of **bodywork** and psychotherapy that promotes healing by bringing a person's mind, body, spirit, and emotions into the healing process. Ilana Rubenfeld, who developed this healing method, realized the intimate connection among

body, mind, spirit, and emotions while she sought relief from debilitating back pain at the hands of an Alexander Technique teacher and emotional support from a psychiatrist. Her search prompted her to learn not only the **Alexander Technique** but also the **Feldenkrais Method**, **Gestalt therapy**, and hypnosis. Rubenfeld drew on the concepts from these approaches, made modifications, and developed her unique "touch and talk" therapy.

Rubenfeld believes that people change through pleasure rather than through pain and that a sense of safety during treatment is essential. Also key to effective Rubenfeld synergy treatment is that people cannot change unless they become aware of what is occurring at all four levels (body, mind, spirit, and emotions) and are willing to initiate and allow change. Therefore a Synergist (one who practices Rubenfeld Synergy) combines gentle touch, movement, and dialogue to increase people's awareness of where they are holding emotions in the body, and which are causing physical pain or dysfunction. "Client and Synergist meet in a sacred healing space," says Rubenfeld. Visualization, breathing, humor, and posture awareness are often part of the sessions.

ALSO SEE Rosen Method

Ruta (*Ruta graveolens*) is a homeopathic remedy made from rue, also known as the herb of grace. In ancient times, warriors smeared rue on their sword blades to help them feel invulnerable. In the sixteenth and seventeenth centuries, rue branches were spread on jailhouse floors to protect against lice, which carried typhus fever. "Ruta" comes from the Greek *reuo*, which means "to set free."

Today, ruta is used as a first aid remedy for sprains, especially of the knees, ankles, and wrists, as well as for fractures. Ruta also is effective for eyestrain that is characterized by eyes that feel hot, sore, and bruised from overuse. Other symptoms may include a general feeling of bruised soreness, restlessness, and exhaustion. In individuals with chronic or long-term painful tissues and joints,

such as rheumatism, accompanying symptoms may include intense thirst for cold water, nausea and vomiting when eating, and a constant urge to urinate. People best suited for a ruta remedy are usually dissatisfied and tend to "pick fights."

ALSO SEE homeopathy

S

Sage *(Salvia officinalis)* is a perennial evergreen shrub that has been credited with dozens of medicinal uses. Its reputation caused herb authority Varro E. Tyler, Ph.D., to comment that "If one consults enough herbals . . . every sickness known to humanity will be listed as being cured by sage."

Sage's renown began among the ancient Greeks and Romans, who believed it was a memory enhancer and used it to treat epilepsy, chest ailments, and snakebites. Arab physicians credited it with extending life, and the Chinese used it to treat insomnia, depression, gastrointestinal problems, and mental illness. American colonists enlisted sage as a treatment for insomnia, measles, seasickness, and intestinal worms. Today, sage is recommended to soothe sore throat, canker sores, and bleeding gums, and to boost insulin activity in people with diabetes. It is also useful for soothing digestive complaints and treating minor wounds. It is not known exactly why sage has these healing properties, although its ability to soothe sore throat is credited to the presence of tannins.

St. John's Wort *(Hypericum perforatum)* is a yellow-flowering plant that is widely used for its ability to lift mood and provide relief from anxiety, nervous tension, and

restlessness. The supplement needs to be taken daily for several months before its full effects can be experienced. Benefits are usually apparent, however, even after a few weeks of supplementation.

Throughout history, St. John's wort has been used as a topical agent for treatment of wounds and orally for relief of diarrhea, fever, and pain. In recent years, scientists have been investigating its potential use as an antiviral agent against AIDS. These effects may be linked to the presence of flavonoids, tannins, and carotenoids in St. John's wort. One substance in particular, hypericin, a reddish pigment found in the plant's flowers, is believed to be instrumental in the herb's ability to relieve depression, insomnia, and anxiety.

St. John's wort is a common perennial herb found throughout North America and Europe. There are several guesses as to how it acquired its name. One is that it's in honor of St. John the Baptist because, reports Michael Castleman, author of *The Healing Herbs*, early Christians "believed it released its blood-red oil on August 29, the anniversary of the saint's beheading."

Saw Palmetto (saw pal-MET-to) is a palm tree, native to the southeastern United States and parts of the Caribbean, that produces red berries that are effective in treating prostate enlargement and urinary problems. The berries contain a substance that blocks the effects of androgens, male sex hormones that may cause the prostate to enlarge.

In the Caribbean, saw palmetto has been used as a mild aphrodisiac. Throughout Europe, saw palmetto remedies are widely prescribed for prostate problems, but in the United States the Food and Drug Administration (FDA) has banned any labeling that makes that claim. Many U.S. physicians, however, recommend the herb, which should be taken only under a doctor's supervision.

Selenium (suh-LEE-nee-um) is an essential trace mineral that was identified in the 1960s. It is a potent

antioxidant, immune system booster, and cancer fighter. Its primary function in the body is to work with the anti-oxidant enzyme glutathione peroxidase, which protects red blood cells and their membranes against free radical damage.

Selenium's cancer-fighting activity may be associated with several factors. People who live in areas where the soil is rich in selenium and people who eat selenium-rich foods both have a low incidence of cancer. Scientists also find that blood levels of selenium are low in people who have cancer of the breast, stomach, intestine, colon, bladder and genital tract, and that people with low selenium levels have a twofold greater risk of having cancer than do people who have sufficient levels of selenium.

Selenium's antioxidant properties also may be a factor in its anticancer effects. In this case selenium works closely with vitamin E to protect cell membranes from free radical damage, which can cause abnormal cell growth and function. Selenium also detoxifies two cancer-causing minerals, cadmium and mercury.

Some experts suggest that selenium supplements may help people with asthma, who often have low levels of selenium. Low blood levels of selenium are also a risk factor for heart disease and atherosclerosis. It is believed selenium protects the blood vessel walls from free-radical damage, a process that prompts the development of heart disease and atherosclerosis.

Selenium also may have a role in causing or aggravating the symptoms of anemia. Selenium supplements given to animals with low levels of the mineral have corrected the anemia. Its effectiveness in regulating the inflammation associated with rheumatoid arthritis is still unknown. Scientists have also found that women with low blood levels of selenium have a greater risk for development of fibrocystic breast disease than women with adequate levels.

Self-Hypnosis see hypnotherapy

Sensory Awareness Therapy, also known as sensory reeducation or conscious sensing, is a technique whereby people increase their perception, awareness, and appreciation of their experiences beyond an intellectual understanding. It was developed by Elsa Gindler (1885-1961) in Germany and brought to the United States by one of her students, Charlotte Selver, who first used the term "sensory awareness" to explain the technique.

Sensory Awareness is an unstructured method in that the only "course" to follow is that of inquiry. Those who teach Sensory Awareness use suggested sensory experiments that allow participants to increase their awareness of sensations that involve movement, both internal and external. Students are taught "quiet alertness," which is a conscious awareness of how and where tension and stress exist in the body. With awareness comes the opportunity to change, and the premise of this method is that the body will change if people let it assert its needs. When energy that was suppressed or held in the body is finally released, people report feeling lighter, more energetic, and more satisfied with themselves.

Sensory Awareness therapy is credited with improved posture, easier breathing, positive attitude changes, and enhanced balance, flexibility, and coordination.

Sepia (SEE-pee-ah) (*Sepia officinalis*) is a homeopathic remedy derived from the ink sac of the cuttlefish. It is a popular remedy for menstrual and menopausal problems, as it may relieve sadness, depression, and feelings of discontent in women with premenstrual syndrome. Sepia is indicated in women who have a sallow look, sweat profusely, crave sweets and pickles, and feel chilly. Women with morning sickness respond particularly well to sepia, although it should be taken under a professional's guidance. Symptoms are generally worse for drafts and cold and better for warmth. Sepia is also indicated for people with backache and weakness in the small of the back, throbbing headache, and violent coughing.

The sepia personality is characterized by women who

appear unemotional, but may suddenly weep for no apparent reason. Detached, unemotional men also may respond to sepia. Physically, individuals who are tall and lean with soft facial features, dark hair, and a yellow complexion respond best to sepia.

ALSO SEE homeopathy

Serotonin is a hormone that occurs naturally in the brain and which helps regulate the transmission of nerve impulses in that organ. This function makes serotonin a key player in controlling behavior, mood, and satiety. Therefore, serotonin levels are important when diagnosing and treating depression, obesity, eating disorders, and premenstrual syndrome.

One way the body responds to prolonged stress is to signal the brain that it needs more serotonin. In order to produce it, the body requires the amino acid **tryptophan**. To get tryptophan, the brain sends out a signal that tells the body to consume something starchy or sweet. Once the food is eaten, the tryptophan travels to the brain, where serotonin production begins. The rise in serotonin results in a decrease in stress and relief from associated symptoms, such as overeating, mood swings, and depression.

There are many conventional drugs on the market that affect serotonin levels, including Prozac and Zoloft. Natural ways to impact serotonin levels include stress reduction, diet, nutritional supplementation, and exercise.

Shamanism is the use of the spiritual world for the purpose of healing the sick. The spirits are accessed through shamans—individuals who possess the ability to enter a trance or dream state of altered consciousness and communicate with the spirit world. They also reportedly have the ability to foretell the future, dispel evil spirits, and interpret dreams. Shamans often use herbal medicine and various rituals to enter the dream state and to effect cures for those seeking their help.

Common rituals used by shamans to enter an altered state

of consciousness include rattling, chanting, dancing, drumming, and taking natural hallucinogenics. Shamanism is practiced throughout the world, including the United States, where it is found primarily among Native Americans (medicine men and medicine women); India (yogis and holy men); Africa (witch doctors and sangomas); and Europe (witches and wizards). In Korea, all shamans are female.

Shark Cartilage is a supplement made from the translucent elastic tissue of the shark; some researchers claim it can prevent and inhibit cancer cell growth.

Cartilage is a substance that is found in the skeletons of vertebrates that acts as a connective tissue. In humans, cartilage is perhaps most apparent in the nose, ear, and Adam's apple. Cartilage is a unique tissue in that it does not use nerves, blood vessels, or the lymphatic system to perform its functions. Therefore, cartilage does not receive its nutrients through the blood or lymphatic fluid. This unusual characteristic may be a reason cartilage seems to inhibit the formation of malignant tumors.

In 1983, two researchers showed that shark cartilage contains a substance that significantly inhibits the development of blood vessels (angiogenesis) that nourish solid tumors. In another study completed near the same time, researchers at Harvard University Medical School found that the development of tumor-based cancers and metastasis could be prevented if angiogenesis could be eliminated. These findings resulted in increased interest in the use of shark cartilage for the prevention and treatment of cancer. As yet, scientists have not identified the components in shark cartilage that are responsible for this effect. It is known, however, that shark cartilage draws in oxygen and nutrients from its surface and contains proteins that stop the development of new blood vessels. In addition to its possible cancer-preventing effect, shark cartilage has also been credited with reversing osteoporosis and causing psoriasis patches to fade.

SHEN is an acryonm for Specific Human Energy Nexus, a new approach to healing through energy work. Many of its concepts are based on **therapeutic touch** and **polarity therapy** and are similar to several more energy and body-work therapies, yet SHEN differs from these and other energy work therapies in that it deals *only* with emotions as they are held in the body.

SHEN is based on the premise that emotional health is the foundation of our physical, psychological, and spiritual health. Emotions are intimately associated with physical complaints, and unresolved emotional issues can severely compromise the immune system. Repressed emotional "baggage" can manifest as headache and migraine, ulcers, diarrhea, PMS, heart disease, hypertension, chronic pain, stress disorders, insomnia, depression, phobias, alcoholism, drug dependency, low self-esteem, loss of sexual interest, and eating disorders. SHEN releases the painful or negative emotions that are locked in the body and allows people to regain emotional health and well-being.

SHEN was developed by Richard Pavek, a scientist who became interested in the body's bioenergy field while attending an energy workshop in the 1970s. His subsequent research led him to create SHEN Physio-Emotional Release Therapy, which is based on the following concepts: emotions are vibrating sites deep within the body's energy field, inside the physical body; the physical body contracts when it experiences painful, negative emotions and relaxes when it feels pleasurable ones; and unconscious contractions prevent the organs in the region from functioning properly and trap the painful emotions inside. The natural tendency of the body to contract around painful emotions, which Pavek calls the Auto Contractile Pain Response, causes people to bury emotions and hold them unconsciously, which leads to chronic contraction. This consumes a lot of energy and can lead to the disorders mentioned above.

During a typical SHEN session, practitioners use a featherlight touch to scan the body and identify where energy is blocked. Once the sites have been found, practitioners move energy, or **chi**, from their hands through the recipient, and the flow of concentrated energy between the two individuals breaks up the contractions and restores the body's normal energy flow. Very often clients experience an emotional release as repressed feelings come to the surface.

Shiatsu (shee-AHT-soo) is a form of Oriental massage that originated in ancient China, was introduced into Japan, and then gradually evolved into its present form. Today it consists primarily of acupressure and massage along with some elements of osteopathy and other healing therapies. A shiatsu treatment is designed to balance the entire body and promote the body's natural tendency to heal itself.

"Shiatsu" means "finger pressure," and it involves application of pressure to specific **acupoints** along the various **meridians** or channels that run through the body. Pressure is applied using fingertips, knuckles, elbows, thumbs, knees, or feet and tends to be sustained and static rather than moving. Acupressure is usually interspersed with stretches designed to release muscular tension and enhance relaxation. Gentle massage is also used to increase muscle flexibility and improve joint mobility.

Shiatsu helps reduce stress, boosts energy level, promotes digestion, enhances concentration and mental functioning, and calms the nervous system. Additional benefits include better posture, improved self-esteem and well-being, and relief of back and neck pain.

About 1,000 years ago, **Chinese medicine** was introduced to the Japanese, including a massage technique called **amma**. At the turn of the twentieth century, the Japanese government tried to regulate and license amma because the authorities believed it was losing its therapeutic focus. Some practitioners, however, revitalized amma, stressed its healing qualities, and renamed it shiatsu.

Shiatsu gained recognition in the United States in the 1970s soon after President Richard Nixon returned from China and interest in acupuncture and bodywork was piqued. Wataru Ohashi, who went on to develop his own style of shiatsu, was the individual most responsible for bringing shiatsu to the States.

Shiatsu exists in several forms, including Zen shiatsu and ashiatsu. Zen shiatsu incorporates stretches that help release blockages of **chi** along the meridians. In the Orient, stretching as a therapy is even older than acupuncture and is used to increase flexibility and range of motion as well as strengthen muscles. Ashiatsu, also known as barefoot shiatsu, is a form first practiced by Buddhist monks. It uses the feet and hands to apply rhythmic pressure to regulate nerve function, strengthen the body's immune system, flush out toxins, improve circulation, and make joints more flexible. Ashiatsu practitioners consider the client's breathing patterns, emotional state, lifestyle, and dietary preferences to determine the best treatment to give.

Shiitake (shee-TAH-kee) is a medicinal **mushroom** grown in both Asia and the United States, where it is often called Black Forest mushroom. Shiitake mushrooms have both nutritional and therapeutic value, as they are a rich source of many nutrients (especially **vitamins** B1, B2, B6, and B12, riboflavin, and niacin) and contain many substances known for their healing powers.

Shiitake's medicinal value is attributed to some of the many compounds it contains. Polysaccharides make shiitake useful in fighting tumors, bacteria, and viruses by boosting the immune system. It also has been suggested as a treatment for AIDS, and preliminary test results indicate it may possess anticancer properties as well. Researchers have isolated an **amino acid** called eritadenin from shiitake, which is believed to lower cholesterol levels.
ALSO SEE reishi

Skullcap (*Scutellaria lateriflora*) is sometimes called blue skullcap because of its characteristic blue flowers. This herb, found in meadows and by streams, was once known as mad-dog weed, which refers to its use in past centuries to treat rabies and insanity.

Today, skullcap is used primarily for its sedative properties and for its ability to soothe muscular incoordination. The leaves of skullcap are used to prepare remedies to treat headache, insomnia, epilepsy, teething, neuralgia, restlessness, hypertension, and nervous disorders.

Slippery Elm Bark, taken from the inner bark of the slippery elm tree, was long honored by the Native Americans as a treatment for wounds, stomach ache, sore throat, cough, and infant colic. After Dutch elm disease was introduced into the United States and nearly eliminated our elm forests, this herb became more difficult to get.

Slippery elm bark contains a mucilage—a mucus-like substance—that can soothe and coat the throat and stomach. This substance consists of a polysaccharide, a type of sugar, that appears to hold healing qualities. Slippery elm bark is available in throat lozenges and as a powder or tea. To treat wounds, bedsores, burns, boils, diaper rash, and damaged tissues, the powder can be mixed with water to make a paste.

Sound Therapy is an ancient healing method based on the theory that because everything in the universe is a form of energy and is in a constant state of vibration, changes in vibrations, or frequency, can affect physical and emotional states of being. Sound therapy has been, and continues to be, practiced in cultures around the world, often in the form of music or song. Tibetan monks, for example, still use chanting to treat illness, and Native American tribes have used drumming and chanting ceremonies extensively for both physical and emotional ailments.

Although the sound therapy traditions practiced over the millennia continue to be used, variations and modern technology have infiltrated the field. Modern sound therapists believe there is a natural note or vibration that corresponds to each part of the human body. An affected or diseased portion of the body is said to be out of sync or vibrating at a frequency that is not in harmony with the body. Therefore, to promote healing, therapists direct specific sound waves to the affected body part to restore balance and, with it, health. Sound waves may be in the form of voice, musical instruments, or synthesized sound from special machines that transmit vibrations. This latter technique is commonly known as Cymatics.

A simple form of sound therapy that involves the voice is toning, which is the use of sound to create vibrations in the body. Perhaps the most common form of vocal toning is the sound many people use during meditation, the "om." The continuous vocalization of this or another long sound is believed to have a positive calming effect on the mind and body. Experts attribute this benefit to the fact that the vagus nerve, a long nerve that passes through the larynx and many internal organs, is one of the cranial nerves that is affected by sound.

Sound therapy is reported useful in the treatment of conditions such as arthritis, back and neck pain, sports injuries, fractures, rheumatism, and various types of soft-tissue damage. It also has been successful in working with mentally and physically handicapped children and adults. Many sound therapists believe this therapeutic approach is effective in easing any physical or mental condition associated with tension or stress.

ALSO SEE music therapy; light therapy

Spirulina (spee-roo-LEE-nah) is a freshwater, one-celled blue-green microalgae that thrives in high-salt alkaline waters in subtropical areas. It has been around for 3.6 billion years and has been used as a food source for at least four centuries, although it is relatively new to American shelves. Use of spirulina can be traced to various African tribes, who scooped the scum from their lakes, dried it and ground it into flour, and made cakes. Spirulina is also harvested from Lake Texcoco near Mexico City, a tradition that has continued since at least the early sixteenth century when the Aztecs used it as a primary food source.

Spirulina is high in protein (about 60 percent plus) and supplies 100 percent of the Recommended Daily Allowance of **amino acids**. It is also high in iron and many vitamins and minerals, and contains only 5 percent fat. It is often touted as a "miracle" supplement because of its high nutritional levels. However, many experts believe that while spirulina's high protein content may make it an excellent food source for malnourished people in developing countries, it is unnecessary for Americans, who typically ingest too much protein. Both spirulina and another algae, chlorella, are available as tablets or powders and are very expensive.

Spirulina and other algae products readily absorb toxic substances such as heavy metals (e.g., mercury and lead) and nitrates from fertilizers. Consumers are urged to buy only supplements from reputable manufacturers.

Sports Massage is a specialized form of Swedish massage developed specifically for athletes, dancers, and those who wish to improve the body's peak efficiency. It can be done before physical activity to help prevent injuries and pain as well as improve performance. After activity is over, sports massage helps the body eliminate toxins such as lactic acid, and restores range of motion and muscle tone.

Swedish Massage is a therapeutic series of strokes applied to the body to induce relaxation, increase range of motion, remove toxins from the body, enhance recovery from trauma and stress, and promote circulation. It is believed to be the most commonly performed type of massage in the United States and is the foundation from which traditional Western massage techniques emerged.

Swedish massage was developed by Per Heinrik Ling (1776-1839), who drew upon his research into anatomy and physiology, blood circulation, and Eastern healing practices as he developed this massage approach. It incorporates several primary strokes, including effleurage (gliding), tapotement (tapping), vibration (shaking), petrissage (kneading), and friction (rubbing). These strokes are typically applied with the help of massage oils, which help reduce friction and keep the strokes smooth and flowing.

In addition to feeling good, Swedish massage helps relieve stiff joints and pain associated with muscle tension, strains, sprains, and overuse. Swedish massage also can help reduce recovery time after surgery and prevent or reduce muscle atrophy in individuals who are inactive because of disease, injury, or age. Many people also report emotional and psychological benefits, such as a reduction in anxiety, feelings of well-being and relaxation, increased creativity, and fulfillment of their need for nurturing.
ALSO SEE deep tissue massage; Esalan massage; massage; sports massage

Symphytum (sim-FI-tum) *(Symphytum officinale)* is a homeopathic remedy derived from the herb **comfrey**. Its common name is knitbone because it has been characterized with the ability to heal broken and damaged bone and cartilage. In **homeopathy**, it is a common first aid remedy especially for facilitating recovery from broken bones, trauma to the joints or cartilage, injuries to the eyes, and backache. Because it is used almost exclusively as a shortterm remedy, no psychological profile has been established for its use.

T

Tai Chi Ch'uan (tie jee chew-on) is an ancient Chinese martial arts technique that is often called ''meditation in motion.'' Officially it is known as tai chi ch'uan: *tai* means ''supreme,'' *chi* means ''ultimate,'' and *ch'uan* means "boxing" or "fist." The art of tai chi ch'uan (usually shortened to tai chi) unites mind and body by integrating mental focus, awareness of breathing, and slow, measured, graceful movements. In the United States, tai chi is practiced primarily for health reasons, as it helps relieve stress and anxiety and promotes overall health.

Tai chi brings together the Chinese philosophy of yang (positive) and yin (negative), the eternal opposites. Although its origins are lost, tai chi is believed to have emerged about 3,500 years ago. The first recognizable postures have been attributed to a Chinese monk named Chang san Feng, who lived about 600 years ago.

From their very first tai chi lesson, students train both their bodies and their minds to relax and be in harmony. Often, teachers suggest colorful imagery to help students understand the mental and spiritual aspects of tai chi as they learn the physical movements. The entire experience includes learning how to relax all major muscles and to move without tension and stress while at the same time achieving inner peace, awareness, and calm.

In tai chi, every move is gentle and natural, the way nature designed the body to move. When the positions are done correctly (traditional tai chi includes more than 100 movements; modern, abbreviated forms include twenty-four to forty-eight), the spinal column moves into natural alignment. This allows the internal organs to stay in their proper places and prevents any unnatural internal pressure. Tai chi also strengthens bones. According to tai chi philosophy, the vital energy of those who practice the art accumulates just below the navel. It gradually grows hot and travels throughout the body, clearing blocked energy and opening up joints. The bones become stronger because **chi** condenses inside the bones and forms extra marrow.

The controlled, slow motion characteristic of tai chi builds strength, and strong muscles are less likely to cause pain or allow injury. Tai chi facilitates recovery from injury and eliminates the pain associated with arthritis, rheumatism, back pain, and knee injuries. Even stiff, tense individuals learn to relax and strengthen their bodies without risking injury or stress when they practice tai chi. It is recommended for young children and has proven very beneficial to the elderly.

Tai chi has gained recognition from conventional medical arenas. The National Institute on Aging and the National Institutes of Health have performed studies on tai chi practice in the elderly and find that tai chi can significantly reduce the risk of falls among older people. It also may be beneficial in maintaining gains made by people age seventy years and older who do other balance and strength training therapies.

Taoism (DAU-iz-em) is thought to be the oldest Chinese religion. The word *tao* means "the Way," and for Taoists the way to live is to lead a virtuous life, in complete harmony with nature and the universe. Those who live in that way can hope to attain prosperity and immortality. It was founded by Lao-tzu in the sixth century B.C. Some Taoists practice meditation and use chanting to call upon the spirits for healing purposes.

Tea Tree Oil (*Melaleuca alternifolia*) is a pale yellow oil derived from the leaves of the Australian tea tree. It is an ancient remedy used by the aborigines of eastern Australia to treat cuts, boils, and insect bites.

Tea tree oil is a powerful antibiotic, antiviral, and antifungal that is useful for many types of infections, including athlete's foot, canker sores, and nail infections. It is used to treat burns and, in some hospitals in Switzerland, is even used to control the spread of infection. Because of its healing, soothing nature, tea tree oil is used in many health and beauty products, including soaps, shampoos, and body lotions.

Thai Massage (tie) is a technique that resembles **shiatsu** in that practitioners use their palms, fingers, elbows, forearms, knees, and feet to apply pressure to specific pathways in the body to release any blocked energy and to restore unhindered flow of the vital force. Rather than follow the Chinese system of **meridians**, however, Thai massage practitioners more closely follow the Hindu energetic system of *nadis*, which is similar to the Chinese system in concept. This tradition has been carried down by practitioners in Thai Buddhist temples for more than 2,500 years and has its roots in ancient yoga practices.

Thai massage therapists often incorporate deep, passive stretching exercises during massage sessions, which increase range of motion, raise energy levels, and stimulate the client's flow of **chi**. Thai massage is effective in people who have long-term chronic aches and pains and neuromuscular conditions.

ALSO SEE massage

Thalassotherapy (thuh-LAS-oh-THER-uh-pee) is a form of hydrotherapy that utilizes sea water (*thalassa* is Greek for sea) in a variety of ways to improve health and well-being. Thalassotherapy is practiced primarily at spas and resorts where people are treated with sea water massages, underwater jet massage, special circulation showers, water exercises, and other therapeutic treatments. This form of hydrotherapy is credited with many health benefits: relief of stress and fatigue, weight loss, cleansing of the sinuses and respiratory passages, regulation of blood pressure and hormone levels, increase in body metabolism, improved skin and hair quality, and a strengthened cardiovascular system.

Therapeutic Touch is an energy therapy designed to restore balance to the body. It was developed by Dora Kunz, a spiritual healer, and Dolores Krieger, Ph.D., R.N., of New York University. It is based on the principle that illness results when there is an imbalance or blockage in the energy field that surrounds and interpenetrates the body. Practitioners of Therapeutic Touch evaluate a person's energy field and then help to rebalance it. As the energy flow is reestablished, any congestion in the client's energy field is released and the body is free to heal naturally.

Practitioners assess a person's energy field by passing their hands close to, or very lightly touching, the client's body and "feeling" the energy field for congested areas. Such areas may feel like heat, cold, tingling, or other sensations in the practitioner's hands. Once areas of congestion are identified, practitioners focus their own energies to the affected areas to influence the energy flows of their clients. In effect, there is an intermingling of the energy between practitioner and client.

Therapeutic Touch can be effective in relieving headache and other stress-induced pain, speeding recovery from trauma, inducing the relaxation response, and relieving tension and anxiety.

Thyme *(Thymus vulgaris)*, also known as common garden thyme, is a widely cultivated perennial plant that has a long history as a culinary staple and as an herbal remedy. It has powerful antimicrobial and astringent properties and has been used for centuries to treat sore throat, cough, and digestive problems.

Thyme appears to have been used in cooking and as a preservative before its medicinal value was discovered by the ancient Romans, who used it to treat intestinal worms, digestive ailments, and cough. In medieval Germany it was used to treat skin problems, and later it was used during various plagues as an antiseptic. One of thyme oil's active healing ingredients, thymol, was discovered in 1853 by French chemist M. Lallemand. From that time until World War I, thyme was a popular disinfectant and antiseptic. World War I brought a dramatic increase in demand for thymol on the battlefield, but because most of the world's supply of thymol was produced in Germany, the supply to Americans and their allies was scant, and thymol was replaced by more potent antiseptics.

Today thyme is recommended by herbalists for treatment of fever, whooping cough, asthma, dyspepsia, gas, stomach cramps, diarrhea, and suppressed menstruation. When made into a tea and mixed with other herbs such as rosemary, it is effective in the treatment of headache and nervous afflictions, including elimination of nightmares. Thyme's value as an antiseptic, antibacterial, antifungal, expectorant, and digestive aid are attributed to thymol and another active ingredient, carvacol. Thymol is still used commercially in some antiseptic mouthwashes, including Listerine.

Tongue Diagnosis is a diagnostic method widely used in **Chinese medicine**. To a Chinese medicine practitioner, the shape, color, thickness, moisture, and coating on the tongue are all important indicators of the state of health of the internal organs and the general balance of the body. Each organ and **meridian** is represented by a specific area on the tongue. Thus by "reading" the tongue, Chinese medicine practitioners can detect problem areas in the body. ALSO SEE traditional Chinese medicine

Touch for Health is a self-help form of **applied kinesiology** based on the general concept that the body can heal itself if the energy flow is balanced and unhindered. Touch for Health was developed by Dr. John F. Thie, a chiropractor in California, in the 1970s, after he had studied with Dr. George Goodheart, who founded kinesiology. Touch for Health uses muscle testing to locate areas of blocked energy in the muscles and **meridians** in the body. Once identified, practitioners use **acupressure** and **massage** to treat these points. Touch for Health can improve posture, reduce physical and mental pain and tension, and promote well-being. People can learn Touch for Health and treat themselves and others.

Traction is a broad term for a type of therapy in which weights, pulleys, harnesses, gravity, or straps are used to pull the upper and lower parts of the body in opposite directions. Traction is effective for some individuals who have neck or back pain. The amount of weight or other pressure used and the length of time a person is in traction depend on the individual and his or her physical condition.

The basic premise of traction is to stretch the muscles and ligaments, which in turn increases the space between the vertebrae and enlarges the disc spaces. The desired result is relief from disc or spinal alignment problems and their accompanying pain and discomfort. Traction has been used as a treatment modality since the days of Hippocrates, yet physicians still do not agree about how beneficial it is in treating low back pain, or which variation of traction should be used and when.

Traction can be applied in several ways, including the following: light weights applied continuously for several hours; application of heavier weights for up to thirty minutes; intermittent traction that is applied and released every few seconds; autotraction, in which individuals pull on a harness and regulate the amount of traction; manual-mechanical, in which people are strapped to a specially designed divided table and pulled (often used by chiropractors); and **gravity inversion**, which is referred to as autotraction by some health-care professionals. One common gravity inversion technique involves strapping on special boots, which are attached to an overhead bar, allowing you to hang upside down.

Traditional Chinese Medicine (TCM) is a system of medicine that is based on the principles of internal harmony and balance among the organs, between mind and body, and between mind-body and the external environment. It has existed for at least 2,000 years and is the most popular type of **Chinese medicine** practiced in the United States.

The elements associated with TCM include **acupuncture, moxibustion, herbal medicine, acupressure, cupping**, therapeutic exercises, and nutritional guidelines. All of the practices followed in TCM are based on the concept of **chi**, the universal energy or life force, and its movement along the **meridians** that run through the body. The force that regulates chi and all living things, **yin and yang**, also is a foundational force in TCM. The purpose of TCM, in fact, is to maintain a balance of yin-yang. Disease and illness are seen as an imbalance of the two, and any of the abovementioned elements can be used to restore harmony. According to TCM, the body is composed of five basic elements—wind, fire, earth, water, and metal. Good health and well-being depend on all of these elements coexisting in balance. Any one of these elements can be affected by diet, emotions, the seasons, and the external environment; therefore all of these factors are considered by TCM practitioners when they make diagnoses and prescribe treatments.

Trager Approach (TRAY-ger) is a mind-body healing technique that combines two elements: pain-free, hands-on bodywork, called Psychophysical Integration; and simple exercises, called Mentastics (''mental gymnastics''). These two approaches work together to release tension and stress held in various places throughout the body. When the held energy is released, pain, discomfort, and dysfunction disappear.

The Trager Approach was developed by Milton Trager, M.D., who believed that pain and tension begin in the mind and that the nervous system causes the muscles to remain in painful, chronically contracted positions. According to Trager, ''Tight muscles [can] be caused by many things, but the pattern of the tightness is all in the mind.'' Thus Trager sessions involve teaching the client's unconscious (explained below), which is where Trager believes real change occurs.

To eliminate or reduce the client's pain, practitioners ''hook up'' during Psychophysical Integration. Hook-up is a term Trager used to describe the deep meditative state the practitioner enters to access the energy flow around the client. While practitioner and client are ''hooked up,'' the former establishes a deep rapport with the client's unconscious as he or she applies gentle, rhythmic kneading, rocking, stretching, vibrating, and shaking movements to communicate feelings of relaxation, softness, and less pain to the client's mind via the nervous system.

The Mentastics exercises are relaxed, dancelike movements designed to support and reinforce the unconscious messages received during Psychophysical Integration. They are usually taught and performed in a group setting, but clients are encouraged to practice them at home to secure maximum benefit.

The Trager Approach is effective in treating people with degenerative muscular conditions such as polio, multiple sclerosis, and muscular dystrophy; chronic pain conditions such as low back pain; asthma; headache; and emphysema.

Transcendental Meditation (TM) is a meditation technique that was developed in the 1950s specifically for busy individuals who want and need an "abbreviated" version of meditation. TM is the brainchild of an Indian monk named Maharishi Mahesh Yogi, who based it on the concept that people can mentally repeat mantras consisting of short words or phrases to reach a deep state of consciousness and quiet alertness.

The TM technique is a natural, effortless procedure whereby people use mantras to reach the source of all thought, which is transcendental or pure consciousness, and the source of creativity. Some describe the TM process as allowing the mind to flow like a stream into a river, and a river into the ocean, ever increasing in consciousness and awareness. It is typically practiced several times a day, while sitting comfortably with the eyes closed. As the body relaxes, the mind transcends all thoughts and other mental activity and experiences simple awareness, or transcendental consciousness.

More than 500 scientific studies have been conducted on TM. Research shows that TM heals the body, mind, and spirit, as it reduces stress, decreases high blood pressure, increases happiness, stimulates creativity and intelligence, improves memory, raises energy levels, reduces insomnia, increases self-confidence and self-esteem, and reverses biological aging. It is also effective in treating anxiety, depression, asthma, bronchitis, menstrual problems, panic attacks, and phobias. The American Heart Association journal *Hypertension* notes that TM lowers blood pressure and reduces stress-related hormones. TM taught to prisoners has resulted in lower incidences of violence and may be effective in their rehabilitation.

Tryptophan (TRIP-toe-fan), or L-tryptophan, is an amino acid that the brain uses to produce **serotonin**, **melatonin**, and niacin. Its primary role is to regulate the sleep-wake cycle in the brain. Tryptophan also maintains an intimate relationship with zinc and vitamins B3 and B6.

When used alone or with **phenylalanine**, tryptophan is an effective treatment for depression. It is also a safe alternative to sleeping pills. However, currently it is illegal to sell supplements of tryptophan. In the fall of 1989, the FDA recalled tryptophan, stating that it caused a rare and deadly condition called eosinophilia-myalgia syndrome. Although this claim was later found to be untrue, the ban remains. Until it is lifted, you can select foods rich in tryptophan and consume them before retiring to help ensure a good night's sleep. These foods include bananas, dry-roasted sunflower seeds, **spirulina** (excellent source), baked potatoes, and roasted pumpkin.

Tuina (t-WAH-nuh) is a system of manual therapy based on ancient Chinese traditional medicine. "Tuina" means "to push" *(tui)* and "to lift and squeeze" *(na)*. Tuina practitioners facilitate healing by using as many as 365 or more different hand techniques—from gentle and soothing to strong and vigorous—to regulate circulation of blood and **chi**. These techniques include variations of rubbing, shaking, pressing, waving, percussion, and manipulating.

The primary goal of tuina is to prevent disease and to maintain balance and harmony. It has been practiced for more than 2,000 years in China and is gradually making its way to the West. In addition to aiding circulation, tuina helps the body rid itself of toxins, promotes proper organ functioning, and stimulates secretion of endorphins and enkephalins, the body's natural painkillers. Chronic pain, sinus congestion, constipation, and nervous disorders often respond to tuina.

ALSO SEE shiatsu

Turmeric (TER-muh-rik) *(Curcuma longa)*, a tropical spice that belongs to the ginger family, has been used for more than 2,500 years both in cooking and for healing purposes. In the **Ayurvedic medicine** system, it is highly revered as a cleansing herb for the entire body. Generally it is taken to ease menstrual cramps, promote menstruation, purify the blood, and as a stomach and liver tonic. When applied externally, it heals cuts, bruises, boils and skin diseases.

Modern scientific analyses show that turmeric contains substances called curcuminoids, which have antioxidant, anti-inflammatory, antimicrobial, and cancer-preventive properties. Turmeric has demonstrated effectiveness in the treatment of arthritis, liver ailments, intestinal parasites, and as a digestive aid, especially in the digestion of proteins. Investigations continue into its possible use in treating cancer.

Tyrosine (TI-ro-seen) is a nonessential **amino acid** that plays a key role in the manufacture of thyroxin, the hormone that regulates the body's growth and metabolism rate. Tyrosine is manufactured in the body when an enzyme converts **phenylalanine**, another amino acid. Both tyrosine and phenylalanine are precursors (agents that precede the production of another substance) of adrenaline and noradrenaline, two hormones which are important for reducing depression and stress.

Tyrosine is often taken as a supplement, along with

phenylalanine and **vitamins**, to aid in weight loss. This combination can help stimulate the thyroid gland to increase metabolism and help the body use food more efficiently.

Uva Ursi *(Arctostaphylos uva-ursi)*, also known as bearberry, is an evergreen ground-cover plant that grows in northern Europe and North America. The Latin name, *uva ursi*, means "the bear's grape," which may have been given to this herb either because bears love to eat it, or because its unappetizing flavor may only appeal to bears.

Uva ursi has a long history of use, dating back to at least the thirteenth century when it was used by the Welsh "Physicians of Myddfai." It was listed in the London Pharmacopoeia for the first time in 1788, although it was probably used before that time. The Native Americans made a smoking mixture from the leaves and called the plant *kinnikinnik*.

Uva ursi contains a substance called "arbutin," which transforms itself into a potent urinary antiseptic called "hydroquinone" once it reaches the urinary tract. This property makes uva ursi especially effective in the treatment of urinary tract disorders, such as nephritis, cystitis, urethritis, kidney stones, bladder stones, pyelitis (inflammation of the pelvis of the kidney), hematuria (bloody urine), yeast infections, vulvitis, and the pain associated with genital herpes and venereal warts. Women who experience painful menstruation can take uva ursi for relief, as the herb constricts the blood vessels in the lining of the uterus. Uva ursi also is helpful in treating urinary incontinence, diabetes, dysentery, piles, hemorrhoids, gonorrhea, and syphilis. When prepared as a tea, it can be applied as a wash for abrasions, infections, bruises, and contusions.

Because uva ursi has a high level of tannins, it should not be used for more than two to three days, as it will irritate the stomach lining and the kidneys, and the hydroquinone is poisonous.

Valerian (vuh-LAR-ee-en) *(Valeriana officinalis)* is an odorous plant that is generally considered to be one of the most useful relaxing herbs on the market. Its sedative properties have made it the active ingredient in more than 100 over-the-counter sleep aids and tranquilizers in West Germany.

Legend has it that the Pied Piper of Hamelin lured the rats and children out of the village using valerian root. But valerian's tranquilizing properties were well known long before the Pied Piper used this herb. The ancient Greeks and Romans also used it as a diuretic and as an antidote to poisons. In the sixteenth and seventeenth centuries, it was recommended for chest congestion, bruises, convulsions, menstruation, and wounds. The Native Americans used it to treat wounds, and the colonists soon discovered its sedative value.

Today, valerian is most often used as a safe, mild alternative sedative to benzodiazepines, such as Valium. Investigations are underway to determine its effectiveness in treating epilepsy and hypertension.

Vegetarianism (vej-uh-TAR-ee-en-iz-em) is a dietary and lifestyle choice in which people eat foods that are of plant origin and do not consume meat, poultry, or fish, and/or other products from animals, such as eggs, milk and other dairy products. There are three basic types of vegetarians: vegans, who eat only plant-based foods and none of the products named above; ovo-vegetarians, who add eggs to their plant-based diets; and ovo-lacto-vegetarians, who add eggs and dairy products to their plant base. Some people who occasionally eat fish or chicken but basically shun all other meat or animal products call themselves "semivegetarians," although many "pure" vegetarians argue that such people are not vegetarians.

More and more experts in the medical and health care field recognize vegetarianism as the healthiest diet to follow, and many large-scale studies are verifying these beliefs. The dietary link between consumption of animal products, which are laden with fat and cholesterol, and most types of cancer, heart disease, stroke, diabetes, hypertension, gallstones, osteoporosis, and many other diseases has been and continues to be shown in study after study. Well-known physicians, such as John McDougall, M.D., and Dean Ornish, M.D., use vegetarian diet plans in their treatment clinics for diabetes, heart disease, and hypertension. T. Colin Campbell, Ph.D., who conducted the largest study (65,000 people) on vegetarianism, notes that "Humans are basically a vegetarian species, [and] animal foods are not really healthful, and we need to get away from eating them." Vegetarianism has been endorsed by many medical organizations, including the American Dietetic Association.

A vegetarian diet is recommended not only for the above-named conditions but has been shown in some studies to be effective in people who have food sensitivities and in treating multiple sclerosis, asthma, gout, irritable bowel syndrome, arthritis, and systemic lupus erythematosus.

Vegetarianism is not new: it is mentioned in the Bible; Socrates, Galileo, Cicero, Leonardo da Vinci, and many other well-known (and unknown) people were vegetarians; the Hindus have practiced it for millennia, and most Seventh Day Adventists are vegetarian. Traditional Chinese food is considered to be "semivegetarian," as it contains minute amounts of fish or meat.

Vibrational Healing Massage Therapy is a massage form introduced in 1981 by Patricia A. Cramer, who offers it as a quick and simple way to restore vitality and energy to the circulatory, lymphatic, and nervous systems. This massage form evolved out of her experiences with **polarity therapy**, which she studied with Pierre Pannetier, and her background in athletics, dance, **tai chi**, aikido, and **meditation**. Vibrational healing massage greatly complements other forms of **bodywork** such as **Swedish massage**, **Trager Approach**, **reflexology**, and **craniosacral therapy**.

Vibrational healing massage is effective in treating musculoskeletal aches and pains, including neck and back pain, sports injuries, and headache. It also promotes a new awareness in how people move their bodies. This awareness, which Cramer calls The Fluid Body Model, is one in which people become like fluids, rather than solids, and become more conscious of the fluidity of their movements from moment to moment. Many people report feeling energized and more alert after a massage session.
ALSO SEE massage

Vision Therapy (also called vision training) consists of a program of eye exercises that can improve certain vision problems, such as lazy eye (amblyopiea), eyestrain and fatigue, focusing trouble, and crossed eyes (strabismus). Although vision therapy is not useful for most people with nearsightedness (myopia), it can be beneficial if you have the type in which the eye muscles are overly tense or rigid. Glaucoma and cataracts do not respond to vision therapy.

In the early part of the 1900s, a few eyecare professionals questioned whether anything else besides glasses could help people with vision problems. William H. Bates, M.D., an ophthalmologist, actively pursued that curiosity and developed the **Bates Method of Vision Training**, a series of stress-reducing eye exercises. Bates also said that vision was both physical and "mental," but his ideas about the mind-body concept caused most of his colleagues to laugh at him. Still, Dr. Bates put forth his work in a 1940 book entitled *The Bates Method for Better Eyesight without Glasses.*

Since then, interest has grown in vision therapy, and researchers have promoted and modified Bates' original methods. Today's vision therapy involves not only exercising the eye muscles but also retraining the way the brain processes the images it receives. Vision therapy is offered most often by optometrists (individuals trained to treat vision only) and by some ophthalmologists (physicians who perform surgery and dispense medications for eye conditions). The exercises chosen by your practitioner will be specific to your eye problem and must be done daily, often for a minimum of several weeks, before results become evident. Many athletes who need to "keep their eye on the ball"—such as those who play tennis, baseball, handball, and squash—use vision therapy to improve their games. ALSO SEE Bates Method of Vision Training

Visualization Therapy is a healing approach in which people use positive images during meditation to bring about a desired result, such as pain relief, improved circulation, or relief from tension. The art of conjuring up images for healing purposes has been used for thousands of years, and perhaps longer. Most recently, the use of visualization as a therapeutic approach has been explored by Carl Simonton, Stephanie Simonton, Bernard Siegel, M.D., and many others.

During visualization, people enter a very relaxed state and totally focus their attention on an image or images in the mind's eye on which they have chosen to concentrate. Through a process of suggestions and subtle adjustments to the image, people can eliminate any negative factors and allow in positive, healing ones. There are documented cases in which people have used visualization to reduce or eliminate pain associated with tumors, cancer, and arthritis; to eliminate phobias; and to manage various mental conditions such as depression or anxiety. It also eases asthma and other respiratory conditions and is useful during relaxation exercises.

Scientists have a theory as to why visualization works. Visual, auditory, and tactile (touch) imagery are produced in the thinking and language portion of the brain, the cerebral cortex. A special scanning technique called *positron emission tomography (PET)* has shown that brain activity in the cerebral cortex is equal whether people actually experience something or if they only have a vivid picture of it in their minds. Thus the brain sends the same message to the body regardless of whether the image is real or not. The messages sent cause the body's natural relaxation chemicals to rise, which causes heart rate and breathing rate to decrease. As the body enters a state of relaxation, pain thresholds increase. The more vivid the image, the more effective the visualization session will be.

ALSO SEE imagery

Vitamins are organic substances that, in varying small amounts, are needed by the body for normal functioning and to prevent deficiency diseases. There are thirteen vitamins, present in most foods, and if a person's diet contains fresh, nutritious foods, he or she may be receiving the optimal amount of vitamins for health. Most people, however, are usually deficient in one or more vitamins, **minerals**, trace elements, or other nutritional substances and need to supplement their diets. Some vitamin supplements can be used to treat specific symptoms or ailments.

Generally, vitamin supplements should be taken with food, as they can cause stomach upset, heartburn, and other gastric problems. Natural and synthetic vitamins provide essentially the same benefits, although some vitamins may contain ingredients that enhance potency and some brands may contain fillers you wish to avoid, such as talc or gelatin.

Vitamins fall into two categories: water-soluble and fat-soluble. The former are easily eliminated from the body and consist of all B vitamins and vitamin C; the latter (vitamins A, D, E, and K) can accumulate in the body and reach toxic levels in rare cases.

This is not a "how-to" book and so does not give recommended or suggested supplementation levels of vitamins. The accompanying box does, however, provide information on the role of specific vitamins and which symptoms and conditions they may alleviate or cure, or situations in which supplements may be beneficial, if applicable. Consult the Nutritional Therapies sections of the Appendixes for sources of in-depth information.

VITAMINS

Vitamin A (retinol): maintains night vision, development of skin and mucous membranes, builds bones and teeth; an antioxidant and protector against cancer, Beta-carotene is the water-soluble precursor of vitamin A

Vitamin B1 (thiamine): assists in carbohydrate metabolism, promotes nerve function; is destroyed by alcohol—supplement if alcohol is consumed frequently

Vitamin B2 (riboflavin): helps release energy from food; promotes vision and healthy skin

Vitamin B3 (niacin): assists carbohydrate metabolism, promotes healthy skin and nerves; supplements may help people with Raynaud's disease or cold extremities, or smokers who have leg cramps

Vitamin B6 (pyridoxine): assists metabolism of protein, fat, and carbohydrates; supplement may relieve premenstrual syndrome, depression, arthritis, and nerve compression injuries; protects immunity

Vitamin B12 (cyanocobalamin): promotes development of red blood cells and nerve tissue; is usually deficient in people who do not eat any animal products

Folic acid (folacin): promotes development of red blood cells; may reverse mild to moderate cervical dysplasia; prevents birth defects

Pantothenic acid: assists in metabolism of protein, fat, and carbohydrates

Biotin: important in metabolism of protein, carbohydrates, and fat

Vitamin C: strengthens blood vessels, assists in iron absorption, facilitates healing; an antioxidant, boosts the immune system, fights cancer; supplement if you have cancer, chronic or infectious disease, or any serious illness; or if exposed to excessive stress, smoking, drugs, alcohol, or carcinogenic foods

Vitamin D: promotes strong bones and teeth; supplement only if not exposed to even minimal sunlight

Vitamin E: prevents destruction of vitamins A and C, fatty acids, and cell membranes; an antioxidant and anticoagulant; helpful in treating premenstrual syndrome, painful menstruation, and wound healing

Vitamin K: facilitates blood clotting

Watsu (WAT-soo) is a form of aquatic bodywork, or water **shiatsu**, created by Harold Dull in the early 1980s. It is a unique therapy in that it provides not only a massage but also an experience that causes healing at the physical, emotional, mental, and spiritual levels. This healing can occur not only for the receiver of watsu, but also for the giver.

Harold Dull's inspiration for inventing watsu began when he traveled to Japan in the late 1970s to study Zen shiatsu, a form of **massage** that emphasizes stretching, range of motion, and **acupoint** work. Harold discovered that these practices can be made more effective if people do stretching exercises while they float in warm water. Watsuers (those who practice watsu) support and rock a client's body while stretching the limbs and keeping the body in continual motion. This continuous, graceful movement does not allow resistance to develop, and the potential for pain is greatly reduced. Without pain, clients are encouraged to move more and farther than they might try out of the water.

The warm water and the support it provides helps remove the weight from the vertebrae and spine and relax the muscles. Freeing of the spine is key to every watsu treatment, because it allows the body's healing energy to be released and with it physical and emotional stress and tension. Once the muscles are relaxed, circulation improves and carries away toxins, which helps reduce fatigue and pain. Watsu practitioners find that even people who are not flexible enough to be placed into some of the more complex watsu stretches greatly benefit from gentle rocking and stretching in the water.

Watsu can be easily learned by people who have no previous experience in **bodywork**, and those who have experienced other therapies often incorporate techniques from other bodywork therapies into their watsu sessions. When people first begin taking watsu sessions, most watsuers start with a set series of movements and then move on to more "free form" work as the clients advance. People are also encouraged to develop their own movements that respond to their unique needs.

Watsu provides relief to people with acute and chronic muscle aches and pains, including neck and lower back pain, headache, and sports injuries. According to watsu practitioners, it also benefits the emotional, psychological, and spiritual aspects of those who receive treatments, because of the trust clients must place in the hands of the watsuer to hold and nurture them in the water. Each person who experiences watsu carries something different away from the sessions. Some people say they get an increased awareness of where tension is stored in the body; some say they overcome the fear of water. For others, it may even allow them to re-experience birth.

Wheat Grass refers to the young leaves of the grain-producing wheat plant. Wheat grass is just one in a group of what are known as "cereal grasses," which includes barley, oats, kamut, millet, and rye. The cereal grasses are part of a larger group of "green superfoods," which also includes spirulina and various microalgaes.

Scientists became interested in the cereal grasses in the 1930s in an effort to improve the nutritional value of animal feed. They discovered that wheat and other grasses fed to livestock resulted in a dramatic increase in egg and milk production. The factors responsible for this increase are believed to be the intricate balance of enzymes, antioxidants, and other nutrients in wheat grass and other cereal grasses.

The step from animal to human consumption was first made in the 1960s by Dr. Ann Wigmore, who had a case of gangrene that nearly made her lose her legs. She saved her legs from amputation by taking wheat grass. Today, wheat grass is available on the market as a concentrated food source, rich in chlorophyll, fiber, calcium, beta-carotene, iron, protein, vitamins C, B12, B6, and K, folic acid, and minerals.

Chlorophyll is one of the most important nutrients in wheat grass, because it is instrumental in healing. It protects against toxins, cleanses the digestive tract, promotes intestinal regularity, and is an excellent wound healer. Wheat grass can be used on the skin for burns, bruises, acne, eczema, poison ivy, and cuts. It is effective in the treatment of hemorrhoids, as a wash for sore eyes, in the mouth for gum problems, and in colonics and enemas.

White Willow *(Salix alba)* is often referred to as the herbal equivalent of aspirin, but without the side effects. In fact, white willow does cause mild stomach distress in a small number of users, but not to the degree, magnitude, or prevalence associated with aspirin use.

The leaves and bark are used in herbal remedies to treat fever, headache, and the pain characteristic of arthritis, rheumatism, sciatica, and neuralgia. White willow contains salacin, which metabolizes to acetylsalicylic acid, or "aspirin," the source of its painkilling abilities.

Wild Yam *(Discorea villousa)* is a plant that contains a natural progesterone substance. Commonly referred to by its Latin name discorea, it is perhaps best known for relieving symptoms of menstruation and menopause. This is not a recent discovery, however. Folk herbalists have used wild yam since the eighteenth century to treat menstrual cramps and problems related to childbirth.

In 1936, Japanese scientists in Mexico discovered that a specific type of wild yam contains a chemical, called diosgenin, that is very similar to progesterone. Diosgenin is used in the manufacture of contraceptive pills, and more than 200 million prescriptions sold each year contain this derivative.

This natural progesterone is far superior to synthetic progesterone, says John Lee, M.D., an expert on progesterone and menopause, because the latter "is not progesterone. The pharmaceutical companies alter the molecular structure so it no longer fits into the biochemical machinery of the body." Wild yam does not cause masculinization or fluid retention, as does synthetic progesterone, nor does it increase women's risk of breast or endometrial cancers, or cardiovascular disease. In fact, it is believed to stimulate production of **DHEA**, which can help protect against heart disease. Dr. Lee also claims that according to his bone density studies, wild yam can increase bone density by 10 percent in the first six to twelve months of use.

Wild yam is believed to provide progesterone that is superior to synthetic progesterone because the substance taken from wild yam is nearly identical to what the body produces. Wild yam is available as a cream, capsule, oil, and tablet either over the counter or from a physician. The cream and oil formulas are the most effective because they are absorbed through the skin and into the bloodstream. Capsules and tablets are broken down by stomach acids before they are absorbed into the blood. When buying natural progesterone, be sure the label says it contains progesterone derived from wild yam or a derivative.

Witch Hazel *(Hamamelis virginiana)*, also known as winterbloom and snapping hazelnut, is the liquid extract produced from the leaves and bark of this bushy herb, which grows all over the eastern United States. It is a staple healing herb in many homes: more than one million gallons of witch hazel are sold in the United States each year. Because it has anti-inflammatory, antiseptic, and astringent properties, it is effective for external treatment of hemorrhoids, insect bites, and skin irritation.

The "witch" in witch hazel can be traced back to medieval Middle English, when the word "witch" was spelled *wych* or *wyche* and meant "flexible." This refers to the extreme pliability of witch hazel branches. "Hazel" refers to the plant's resemblance to the common hazelnut.

Native Americans used witch hazel topically to treat cuts, insect bites, aching muscles and joints, and sore backs. They also brewed a witch hazel tea to treat colds, sore throat, and menstrual pain and to eliminate internal bleeding and miscarriage. When colonist Theron T. Pond of Utica, New York, heard about witch hazel's healing properties in the 1840s, he marketed it as Pond's Golden Treasure and later changed the name to Pond's Extract. The original manufactured product had a high level of tannins, which give witch hazel its potent astringent action. Modern processing methods eliminate the tannins, but the remaining decoction reportedly has other elements that give witch hazel its antiseptic, anesthetic, astringent, and anti-inflammatory properties. Contemporary herbalists recommend using witch hazel decoctions made from the bark, which contains tannins.

Witch hazel continues to be widely used for cuts, bruises, burns, inflammation, scalds, and hemorrhoids. It is effective as a gargle for sore throat.

Y

Yerba Santa *(Eriodictyon californicum)*, also called honey herb and mountain balm, is an herb most commonly used for upper respiratory congestion. It is an aromatic evergreen shrub that grows in the mountains of Oregon, California, and northern Mexico. For centuries, the Indians smoked or chewed the leaves to relieve colds and symptoms of asthma. These uses were then passed along to the Spanish missionaries and settlers.

Today yerba santa is still used to treat the spasm of asthma and for chronic bronchitis, laryngitis, cough, sore throat, and fever. It is usually taken as a tea or a syrup.

Yin and Yang is the Chinese philosophy that is the basis for all life and the interdependence of all things. Yin and Yang are opposite yet complementary forces that exist in all of nature and must be in balance for harmony, health, and well-being to be achieved. The theory of yin and yang first appeared during the Chinese Zhou dynasty (1000-770 B.C.). Yang literally means "sunny side of the mountain" and is the male force. It manifests as light, noise, activity, birth, warmth, and form. Yin literally means "shady side of the mountain" and is the female force. Its qualities include coldness, darkness, weakness, and hollowness.

When a person's yin and yang are out of balance, he or she is out of health or in a state of dis-ease. Symptoms such as high fever, abdominal bloating, and headache are signs of excess yang, while chronic fatigue, cold hands and feet, and pale complexion are signs of excess yin. In Chinese medicine, practitioners offer treatments that will restore the balance of yin and yang. The Chinese have identified the

yin and yang qualities of plants and foods and thus can prescribe specific herbs and foods to treat particular conditions and symptoms. To help eliminate fever, for example, yin foods such as mung sprouts, cucumber, potatoes, and summer squash are recommended. To treat cold hands and feet, yang foods, which are warm or hot, such as garlic, parsnips, onions, and scallions, are suggested.
ALSO SEE traditional Chinese medicine

Yoga literally means "union" or "yoking" and is an ancient practice (believed to be about 5,000 years old) developed to integrate and balance the body and mind and create a calm, balanced state of being. The practice is based on the union of the self—mind, body, and spirit—with a higher consciousness. According to yogic philosophy, these three elements cannot be separated, and as humans we are linked with all things, living and inanimate.

Yoga originated among the Hindus of India and has spread throughout the world. Though there are many different types of yoga, the most common ones incorporate stretching movements (called *asanas*), meditation, spiritual enlightenment, and breathing techniques (see box). When yoga is used as therapy, certain positions and postures are usually recommended to facilitate healing. There are hundreds of asanas and variations.

Yoga can be used to successfully treat backache, arthritis, rheumatism, stress and stress-related disorders, high blood pressure, circulatory problems, fatigue, insomnia, anxiety, depression, and digestive disorders. Yoga works simultaneously on the mind and body and gradually strengthens muscles, increases flexibility, and improves stamina. It trains the body to remain quiet and relaxed and to create internal harmony. The overall result of practicing yoga is a sense of well-being and relaxation, flexibility and strength.
ALSO SEE Acu-Yoga

SOME TRADITIONAL FORMS OF YOGA

Hatha Yoga: emphasizes physical positions or asanas and breathing control

Raja Yoga: primarily focuses on meditation

Ashtanga Yoga: combines Hatha and Raja and links the difficult Hatha positions into a flowing movement while integrating the mind to control breathing

Kundalini Yoga: traditionally called the "coiled serpent" that resides at the base of the spine; those who practice Kundalini strive to awaken the serpent (energy) and move it up the spine to the head, a process that activates the chakras

Tantric Yoga: based on Kundalini and works with the chakras; one part of Tantric yoga focuses on awakening sexual pleasure

Yohimbe *(Pausinystalia yohimbe)* is a tree that grows in tropical West Africa. When the plant is made into a tea or is smoked, it gives off yohimbine, which is an alkaloidal salt that is used in prescriptions to enhance sexual performance.

People who take yohimbine report tingling sensations along the spine and in the genitals. Yohimbine works by dilating the blood vessels of the skin and mucous membranes. This results in a drop in blood pressure and an increase in the amount of blood to the sex organs. While this combination of events may increase sexual desire in some people, it may cause temporary impotence in individuals who have low blood pressure.

Yohimbe bark and extracts are available over-the-counter

in health food stores, where people buy it to treat impotence, high blood pressure, arteriosclerosis, angina pectoris, or for use as a local anesthetic. Yohimbe can cause hallucinations, psychosis, and anxiety reactions.

Zen Therapy is a system of spiritual practices and methods based on Buddhist beliefs and philosophy. Though today Zen is practiced primarily in Japan, it originated in India in the sixth century B.C. and wasn't embraced by the Japanese until the twelfth century.

Zen therapy consists of sitting **meditation** *(za-zen)*, which is practiced daily; prolonged meditation that can last for hours or days *(sesshin)*, and reading of Zen writings as a way to enlighten the mind and encourage new ways of thinking. The ultimate goal of Zen therapy is self-enlightenment. The primary focus of Zen is living in the present moment. This is similar to the concept of **mindfulness**. Zen is a deeply personal and spiritual discipline that can result in increased insight, self-awareness, and self-discovery. It is a way of being and living.

Zero Balancing is a form of **bodywork** that incorporates both structural and energetic balancing and concepts from Eastern energy systems and Western bodywork techniques. It was developed in 1975 by Fritz Frederick Smith, M.D., who also practiced osteopathy and acupuncture. Zero balancing is based on the fact that all sentient beings have both a physical and spiritual body. When one body gets injured or out of balance, it affects the whole body. Zero balancing returns both bodies to a state of harmony.

Zero balancing uses a combination of gentle holds, gently applied traction, and sustained stretching positions to affect the energy flow and bring it back to balance. The result is a sense of stillness that leaves clients feeling relaxed, alert, centered, and open. This technique is said to begin a process of energetic integration that continues beyond the session. It allows deeply seated, unconscious tension and stress to be released and may set the stage for long-term patterns of positive behavioral change.

Zinc is an essential mineral that plays a critical role in metabolic processes, synthesis of DNA and RNA, normal growth and development, and cell reproduction. It also is a powerful **antioxidant** and facilitates wound healing. Food sources include milk, sesame and sunflower seeds, soybeans, wheat bran and germ, and whole grain foods.

Zinc appears to be instrumental in the treatment of several medical conditions. Zinc is essential in insulin production, and adequate zinc levels may help restore and maintain normal insulin and blood sugar levels. Results of a University of Kentucky study suggest that zinc supplementation enhances cognitive thinking ability. A zinc deficiency has been linked to schizophrenia and manic depression.

Zinc's antioxidant properties make it useful in combatting viruses, such as herpes simplex, and upper respiratory tract infections. Some women who suffer with premenstrual syndrome have low levels of zinc in their blood, and zinc supplements may relieve their symptoms. Zinc is also used to help relieve the inflammation associated with rheumatoid arthritis and in the treatment of arteriosclerosis.

Organizations and Resources

ACUPRESSURE/ ACUPUNCTURE

Acupressure Institute of America
1533 Shattuck Avenue
Berkeley, CA 94709
(510) 845-1059 or
(800) 442-2232 (outside California)

Acupuncture Research Institute
313 West Andrix Street
Monterey Park, CA 91754

American Academy of Medical Acupuncture
5820 Wilshire Blvd., Suite 500
Los Angeles, CA 90036
(213) 937-5514

American Association of Acupuncture and Oriental Medicine.
433 Front Street
Catasauqua, PA 18032
(610) 433-1433

Chi Nei Tsang Institute
2315 Prince Street
Berkeley, CA 94705
(510) 848-9558

Jin Shin Do Foundation for Bodymind Acupressure
366 California Avenue #16
Palo Alto, CA 94306
(415) 328-1811

Jin Shin Hyutsu Inc.
8719 E. San Alberto
Scottsdale, AZ 85258
(602) 998-9331

Kushi Institute
P.O. Box 7
Becket, MA 01223
(413) 623-5741

The Ohashi Institute
Kinderhook, NY 12106
(518) 758-6879

BODYWORK THERAPIES (MISCELLANEOUS)

American Polarity Therapy
  Association
2888 Bluff Street,
Suite 149
Boulder, CO 80301
(303) 545-2080

The Amma Institute of
  Skilled Touch
1881 Post Street
San Francisco, CA 94115
(415) 564-1103

Biokinesiology Institute
5432 Highway 227
Trail, OR 97541
(503) 878-2080

Institute for Health
  Improvement (Breema)
6076 Claremont Avenue
Oakland, CA 94618
(510) 428-0937

International College of
  Applied Kinesiology
P.O. Box 905
Lawrence, KS 66044
(913) 542-1801

Myofascial Release
  Treatment Center &
  Seminars
Routes 30 and 252
10 S. Leopard Road, Suite 1
Paoli, PA 19301
(610) 644-0136

North American Vodder
  Association of
  Lymphatic Therapy
P.O. Box 861
Chesterland, OH 44026
(216) 729-3258

Therese C. Pfrimmer Intl.
  Association of
  Deep Muscle Therapists,
  Inc.
269 S. Gulph Road
King of Prussia, PA 19406
(800) 484-7773,
  security code 7368

Bonnie Prudden Pain
  Erasure Clinic
7800 E. Speedway
Tucson, AZ 85710
(520) 529-3979

Rolf Institute of Structural
  Integration
205 Canyon Blvd.
Boulder, CO 80302
(800) 530-8875

Rosen Center East (for
  eastern U.S. and Canada)
(800)-484-9832;
  security code 9113
Rosen Center Southwest
  (for Rocky Mountain
  area and southwest)
(505) 982-7149
The Berkeley Center (west
  coast)
(510) 845-6606
Rosen Method Professional
  Association (for all other
  U.S. areas)
(510) 644-4166

The Rubenfeld Center
115 Waverly Place
New York, NY 10011
(212) 254-5100

The Trager Institute
33 Locust
Mill Valley, CA
  94941-2091
(415) 388-2688

Zero Balancing Association
P.O. Box 1727
Capitola, CA 95010
(408) 476-0665

CREATIVE THERAPIES

American Art Therapy
  Association
1202 Allanson Road
Mundelein, IL 60060
(708) 949-6064

American Association of
  Music Therapy
P.O. Box 80012
Valley Forge, PA 19484
(610) 265-4006

American Dance Therapy
  Association
2000 Century Plaza,
  Suite 108
10632 Little Patuxent
  Parkway
Columbia, MD 21044
(410) 997-4040

National Association for
  Music Therapy
8455 Colesville Rd.,
  Suite 930
Silver Spring, MD 20910

EASTERN MEDICINE

American Foundation of
  Traditional Chinese
  Medicine
505 Beach Street
San Francisco, CA 94133
(415) 776-0502

American Institute of
  Vedic Studies
P.O. Box 8357
Santa Fe, NM 87504-8357

American School of
  Ayurvedic Sciences
10025 N.E. Fourth Street
Bellevue, WA 98004
(206) 453-8022

Ayurvedic Institute
1311 Menaul NE, Suite A
Albuquerque, NM 887112
(505) 291-9698

Center for Chinese
  Medicine
230 S. Garfield Avenue
Monterey Park, CA 91754

ENERGY THERAPIES

American Reiki Masters
  Association
P.O. Box 130
Lake City, FL 32056
(904) 744-9638

Feng Shui Institute of
America
P.O. Box 488
Wabasso, FL 32970
(561) 589-9900

Flower Essence Fellowship
Laurel Farm Clinic
17 Carlingcott, Peasedown
St. John
Bath BA2 8AN
Great Britian

Flower Essence Society
P.O. Box 459
Nevada City, CA 95959
(800) 736-9222

Grof Transpersonal
Training
20 Sunnyside Avenue,
Suite A-314
Mill Valley, CA 94941
(415) 383-8779

Homeopathic Academy of
Naturopathic Physicians
14653 South Graves Road
Mulino, OR 97042
(503) 829-7326

Homeopathic Educational
Services
2124 Kittredge Street
Berkeley, CA 94704
(800) 359-9051

International Institute for
Bioenergetic Analysis
144 East Thirty-sixth Street
New York, NY 10016
(212) 532-7742

International Institute of
Reflexology
P.O. Box 12642
St. Petersburg, FL
33733-2642
(813) 343-4811

National Center for
Homeopathy
801 N. Fairfax Street,
Suite 306
Alexandria, VA 22314
(703) 548-7790

Nelson Bach USA Ltd.
Wilmington Technology
Park
100 Research Drive
Wilmington, MA 01887
(508) 988-3833

Nurse Healers—
Professional Associates,
Inc.
P.O. Box 444
Allison Park, PA
15101-0444
(412) 355-8476
Houses Dr. Krieger's
original materials

Omega Institute for
Holistic Studies (color
therapy)
260 Lake Drive
Rhinebeck, NY 12572
(914) 266-4301

Radionics Technique
   Association
P.O. Box 40570
St. Petersburg, FL 33743

The Reiki Alliance
P.O. Box 41
Cataldo, ID 83810
(208) 682-3535

Society for Light
   Treatment and Biological
   Rhythms
10200 West 44th Street,
   Suite 305
Wheat Ridge, CO 80033

Touch for Health
   Association
6955 Fernhill Dr., Suite 5
Malibu, CA 90265
(310) 457-8342 or
(800) 466-8342

HERBS & HERBAL
MEDICINE

American Botanical
   Council
P.O. Box 201660
Austin, TX 78720
(512) 331-8868

American Herb Association
P.O. Box 1673
Nevada City, CA 95959
(530) 265-9552

American Herbalists Guild
P.O. Box 1683
Soquel, CA 95073
(408) 464-2441

Herb Research Foundation
1007 Pearl Street,
   Suite 200
Boulder, CO 80302
(303) 449-2265

MASSAGE

The American Massage
   Therapy Association
820 Davis Street, Suite 100
Evanston, IL 60201-4444
(708) 864-0123

Associated Bodywork &
   Massage Professionals
28677 Buffalo Park Road
Evergreen, CO 80439
(800) 458-2267

Aunty Margaret School of
   Hawaiian Lomilomi
P.O. Box 221
Captain Cook, HI 96704
(808) 323-2416

Esalen Institute
Big Sur, CA 93920
(408) 667-3000

MIND THERAPIES

The Academy for Guided
   Imagery
P.O. Box 2070
Mill Valley, CA 94942
(800) 726-2070

American Association of
Therapeutic Humor
222 South Merrimac #303
St. Louis, MO 63105
(314) 863-6232

American Board of
Hypnotherapy
16842 Von Karman
Avenue,
Suite 475
Irvine, CA 92714
(714) 261-6400

American Society of
Clinical Hypnosis
2200 East Devon Avenue,
Suite 291
Des Plaines, IL 60018
(708) 297-3317

Association for Applied
Psychophysiology and
Biofeedback
10200 West 44th Avenue,
Suite 304
Wheat Ridge, CO 80033

Biofeedback Society of
America
U.C.M.C. c268
4200 E. Ninth Avenue
Denver, CO 80262

Hakomi Integrative
Somatics
P.O. Box 19438
Boulder, CO 80308
(303) 447-3290

Insight Meditation Society
1230 Pleasant Street
Barre, MA 01005
(508) 355-4378

Maharishi International
University
1000 North Fourth Street
Fairfield, IA 52556
(515) 472-5031

National Guild of
Hypnotists
P.O. Box 308
Merrimack, NH 03054

Sensory Awareness
Foundation
1314 Star Route
Muir Beach, CA 94965

Sensory Awareness
Leaders Guild
411 W. 22nd Street
New York, NY 10011

Simonton Cancer Center
P.O. Box 890
Pacific Palisades, CA
90272
(310) 459-4434
(Imagery in cancer
treatment)

MISCELLANEOUS
THERAPIES & METHODS

American Board of
Chelation Therapy
70 W. Huron Street
Chicago, IL 60610
(800) 356-2228

Association for the Study
  of Dreams
P.O. Box 1600
Vienna, VA 22183
(703) 242-8888

International Bio-Oxidative
  Medicine Foundation
P.O. Box 13205
Oklahoma City, OK
73113-1205
(405) 478-IBOM

National Iridology
  Research Association
P.O. Box 31013
Seattle, WA 98103
(206) 282-6604

The Undersea Hyperbaric
  and Medical Society
9650 Rockville Pike
Bethseda, MD 20815
(301) 571-1818

MOVEMENT & POSTURE THERAPIES

(Benjamin System)
  Muscular Therapy
  Institute
122 Rindge Avenue
Cambridge, MA 02140
(800) 543-4740

Body Logic Studio
295 W. 11th Street, 1F
New York, NY 10011
(212) 633-2143

The Body of Knowledge/
  Hellerwork
400 Berry Street
Mt. Shasta, CA 96067

The Feldenkrais Guild
706 S.W. Ellsworth Street
P.O. Box 489
Albany, OR 97321-0142
(503) 926-0981

(Ideokinesis) Irene Dowd
14 E. 4th Street #606
New York, NY 10012

International Association of
  Yoga Therapists
109 Hillside Avenue
Mill Valley, CA 94941
(415) 383-4587

The Kinetic Awareness
  Center
P.O. Box 1050 Cooper
  Station
New York, NY 10276

Mensendieck Academy and
  Enterprises
P.O. Box 9450
Stanford, CA 94309
(415) 851-8184

North American Society of
  Teachers of the
  Alexander Technique
P.O. Box 517
Urbana, IL 61801
(800) 473-0620

The School for Body-Mind
  Centering
189 Pondview Drive
Amherst, MA 01002
(413) 256-8615

Sivananda Yoga
5178 S. Lawrence Blvd.
Montreal, Quebec
H2T 1R8 Canada
(514) 279-3545

Society of Ortho-Bionomy
  International, Inc.
P.O. Box 1974-70
Berkeley, CA 94701
(608) 257-8828

NATUROPATHY

American Association of
  Naturopathic Physicians
2366 Eastlake Avenue E,
Suite 322
Seattle, WA 98102
(206) 323-7610

Homeopathic Academy of
  Naturopathic Physicians
P.O. Box 69565
Portland, OR 97201
(503) 795-0579

Institute for Natural
  Medicine
66½ North State Street
Concord, NH 03301
(603) 225-8844

NUTRITIONAL & SUPPLEMENTAL THERAPIES

American Academy of
  Orthomolecular
  Medicine
900 North Federal
  Highway
Boca Raton, FL 33432
(800) 847-3802

American Natural Hygiene
  Society
P.O. Box 30630
Tampa, FL 33630
(813) 855-6607

Gerson Institute
P.O. Box 430
Bonita, CA 91908
(619) 472-7450

International Academy of
  Nutrition and Preventive
  Medicine
P.O. Box 18433
Asheville, NC 28814
(704) 258-3243

International Association of
  Hygienic Professionals
204 Stambaugh Bldg.
Youngstown, OH 44503
(216) 746-5000

International Macrobiotic
  Shiatsu Society
1122 M Street
Eureka, CA 95501
(707) 445-2290

Vegetarian Education
  Network
P.O. Box 3347
West Chester, PA 19380
(215) 696-VNET

PHYSICAL THERAPIES

American Academy of
  Osteopaths
3500 De Pauw Blvd.,
  Suite 1080
Indianapolis, IN 46268
(317) 879-1881

American Academy of
  Osteopathy
P.O. Box 750
Newark, OH 43055
(614) 349-8701

American Association of
  Naturopathic Physicians
2366 Eastlake Avenue E,
  Suite 322
Seattle, WA 98102
(for hydrotherapy
  information)

The American Chiropractic
  Association (ACA)
1701 Clarendon Blvd.
Arlington, VA 22209
(703) 276-8800

Association for Network
  Chiropractic Spinal
  Analysis
P.O. Box 7682
Longmont, CO 80501
(303) 678-8086

Colorado Cranial Institute
466 Marine Street
Boulder, CO 80302
(303) 447-2760

The Cranial Academy
3500 Depauw Blvd.
Indianapolis, IN 46268
(317) 879-0713

International Chiropractors
  Association
1110 N. Glebe Rd.,
  Suite 1000
Arlington, VA 22201
(703) 528-5000

PSYCHOLOGICAL THERAPIES

American Psychological
  Association
1200 Seventeenth Street
  NW
Washington, DC 20036

SENSORY THERAPIES

Aromatherapy Institute of
  Research
P.O. Box 2354
Fair Oaks, CA 95628
(916) 965-7546

Cambridge Institute for
  Better Vision
65 Wenham Road
Topsfield, MA 01983

National Association for
  Holistic Aromatherapy
219 Carl Street
San Francisco, CA 94117
(415) 564-6785

Optometric Extension
  Program Foundation and
  Vision Extension
2912 S. Daimler Street
Santa Ana, CA 92705
(714) 250-0846

Vision WorkOut
911 West Moano Lane
Reno, NV 89509

Books, Periodicals, and Mail Order Services

ACUPRESSURE/ACUPUNCTURE

BOOKS

Bauer, Cathryn. *Acupressure for Everyone*. New York: Henry Holt, 1991.

Cargill, Marie. *Acupuncture: A Viable Medical Alternative*. Westport, CT.: Praeger, 1994.

Connelly, Dianne M. *Traditional Acupuncture: The Law of the Five Elements*. Columbia, MD: The Centre for Traditional Acupuncture, 1989.

Gach, Michael Reed. *Acupressure's Potent Points: A Guide to Self-Care for Common Ailments*. New York: Bantam Books, 1990.

———. *Acu-Yoga: The Acupressure Stress Management Book*. New York: Japan Publishers, 1981.

Hin, Kuan, Dr. *Chinese Massage and Acupressure*. New York: Bergh Publishing, 1991.

Houston, F.M. *The Healing Benefits of Acupressure*. Rev. ed. Keats, 1994.

Kaptchuk, Ted J. *The Web That Has No Weaver: Understanding Chinese Medicine*. New York: Congdon & Weed, 1983.

Kenyon, Keith, M.D. *Pressure Points: Do-It-Yourself Acupuncture Without Needles*. Arco Publishing, 1984.

Lew, Share K. *TuiNa: Chinese Healing and Acupressure Massage*. 3d ed. Fellowship of the Tao, 1988.

Lundberg, Paul. *The Book of Shiatsu*. London: Gaia Books, 1992.

Marcus, Paul. *Acupuncture: A Patient's Guide*. New York: Thorsons, 1985.

———. *Thorsons Introductory Guide to Acupuncture*. London: Hammersmith, 1991.

Namikoshi, Toru. *Shiatsu Therapy: Theory and Practice*. New York: Japan Publications, 1974.

Ohashi, Wataru. *Do-It-Yourself Shiatsu: How to Perform the Ancient Japanese Art of "Acupuncture Without Needles."* New York: EP Dutton, 1976.

Sohn, Tina. *AMMA Therapy: An Integration of Oriental Medical Principles, Bodywork, Nutrition, and Exercise.* Rochester, VT: Inner Traditions, 1994.

Teeguarden, Iona Marsaa, M.A. *The Joy of Feeling: Bodymind Acupressure.* New York: Japan Publications, 1987.

Thompson, Gerry. *The Shiatsu Manual.* New York: Sterling Publishing, 1994.

Ulett, George A. *Beyond Yin and Yang: How Acupuncture Really Works.* St. Louis, MO: Warren H. Green, 1992.

VIDEOTAPES

Tuini: Chinese Manual Therapy
Chinese Educational Travels, Ltd.
Skokie, IL

Hands-On Health Care catalog
Acupressure Institute
1533 Shattuck Avenue
Berkeley, CA 94709
(various instructional videos)

BODYWORK THERAPIES (MISCELLANEOUS)

BOOKS

Barnes, John F. *Myofascial Release: The Search for Excellence, a Comprehensive Evaluatory and Treatment Approach.* Paoli, PA: Myofascial Release Seminars, 1990.

Benjamin, Ben E. *Are You Tense? The Benjamin System of Muscular Therapy.* New York: Pantheon, 1978.

Juhan, Deane, M.A. *An Introduction to Trager Psychophysical Integration and Mentastics Movement Education.* Mill Valley, CA: Trager Institute, 1989.

Lauterstein, David. "What is Zero-Balancing?" in *Massage Therapy Journal* vol. 33, no. 1 (Winter 1994).

LooyenWork Institute. *LooyenWork 535-Hr Certification Program.* Sausalito, CA: n.d.

Osborne-Sheets, Carole. *Deep Tissue Sculpting.* San Diego: International Professional School of Bodywork, 1990.

Prudden, Bonnie. *Myotherapy: Bonnie Prudden's Guide to Pain-Free Living*. New York: Ballantine Books, 1985.

———. *Pain Erasure: The Bonnie Prudden Way*. New York: Ballantine Books, 1985.

Rolf, Ida P., Ph.D. *Rolfing: Reestablishing the Natural Alignment and Structural Integration of the Human Body for Vitality and Well-Being*. Rochester, VT: Healing Arts Press, 1989.

Rosen, Marion, with Sue Brenner. *The Rosen Method of Movement*. Berkeley, CA: North Atlantic Books, 1991.

Rubenfeld, Ilana. "Gestalt Therapy and the BodyMind: An Overview of the Rubenfeld Synergy Method" in *Gestalt Therapy: Perspectives and Applications*. Ed. Edwin C. Nevis. New York: Gardner Press, 1992.

Schreiber, Jon. *Touching the Mountain: The Self-Breema Handbook: Ancient Exercises for the Modern World*. Oakland: California Health, 1989.

Smith, Fritz Frederick, M.D. *Inner Bridges: A Guide to Energy Movement and Body Structure*. Atlanta, GA: Humanics New Age, 1986.

Teschler, Wilfried. *The Polarity Healing Handbook*. Bath, England (Gateway Books) and San Leandro, California (Interbook, Inc.), 1986.

Trager, Milton, M.D., with Cathy Guadagno. *Trager Mentastics: Movement as a Way to Agelessness*. Barrytown, NY: Station Hill Press, 1987.

Travell, Janet G., M.D., and David G. Simons, M.D. *Myofascial Pain and Dysfunction, the Trigger Point Manual*. Baltimore: Williams & Wilkins, 1983.

VIDEOS

How to Get Started with Bonnie Prudden Myotherapy
Bonnie Prudden
7800 E. Speedway
Tucson, AZ 85710
(520) 529-3979

Trager Institute
21 Locust
Mill Valley, CA 94941
(415) 388-2688
(videos)

CREATIVE THERAPIES

BOOKS

American Art Therapy Association. *Introduction, History, Organization and Therapists (of Art Therapy)*. Mundelein, IL, 1992.

Beaulieu, John, N.D. *Music and Sound in the Healing Arts*. Barrytown, NY: Station Hill Press, 1987.

Maranto, Cheryl D., ed. *The Art and Science of Music Therapy: A Handbook*. Harwood Academic Publishers, 1995.

National Association for Drama Therapy. *Drama Therapy*. New Haven, CT: 1992.

Ornstein, Robert, and David Sobel. *Healthy Pleasures*. Reading, MA: Addison-Wesley, 1989.

EASTERN MEDICINE

BOOKS

Beinfield, Harriet, and Efrem Korngold. *Between Heaven and Earth: A Guide to Chinese Medicine*. New York: Ballantine, 1991.

Bensky, Dan, and Randall Barolet. *Formulas and Strategies*. Seattle: Eastland Press, 1990.

Chen Ze-lin, and Chen Mei-fang. *A Comprehensive Guide to Chinese Herbal Medicine*. Long Beach, CA: Oriental Healing Arts Institute, 1992.

Chopra, Deepak, M.D. *Perfect Health: The Complete Mind/Body Guide*. New York: Harmony Books, 1991.

Frawley, David. *Ayurvedic Healing*. Morson Publishing, 1990.

Kaptchuk, Ted J. *The Web That Has No Weaver: Understanding Chinese Medicine*. New York: Congden and Weed, 1983.

Larre, Claude, and Elisabeth Rochat de la Valle. *Rooted in Spirit: The Heart of Chinese Medicine*. Barrytown, NY: Station Hill Press, 1995.

Lu, Henry C. *Chinese Herbal Cures*. New York: Sterling Publishing Company, 1994.

———. *Chinese System of Food Cures. Prevention and Remedies*. New York: Sterling Publishing Company, 1986.

Reid, Daniel. *Chinese Herbal Medicine*. Boston: Shambala, 1994.

———. *The Complete Book of Chinese Health and Healing*. Boston: Shambala, 1995.

———. *The Handbook of Chinese Healing Herbs*. Boston: Shambala, 1995.

Tang, Stephen, and Martin Palmer. *Chinese Herbal Prescriptions*. London: Rider & Company, 1986.

Tianhan Xue. "Exploring Chinese herbal medicine can foster discovery of better drugs" in *The Scientist* 1996; 10(4):9.

Unschuld, Paul. *Medicine in China: A History of Ideas*. Berkeley: University of California Press, 1985.

Williams, Tom. *Chinese Medicine*. Rockport, MA: Element Books, 1995.

Wiseman, Nigel, and Andrew Ellis. *Fundamentals of Chinese Medicine*, rev. ed. Brookline, MA: Paradigm Publications, 1995.

Yanchi, Liu. *The Essential Book of Traditional Chinese Medicine*. 2 vols. New York: Columbia University Press, 1988.

ENERGY THERAPIES

BOOKS

Baginski, Bodo, and Shalila Sharamon. *Reiki: Universal Life Energy*. Translated by Christopher Baker and Judith Harrison. Mendocino, CA: Life Rhythm, 1988.

Barbara, Ray, Ph.D. *The "Reiki" Factor in the Radiance Technique*. St. Petersburg, FL: Radiance Associates, 1992.

———. *Polarity Therapy Workbook*. New York: BioSonic Enterprises, 1994.

Barnard, Julian, and Martine Barnard. *The Healing Herbs of Edward Bach*. Bath, UK: Ashgrove Press, 1993.

Blackie, Margery G. *The Patient Not the Cure: The Challenge of Homeopathy*. London: Macdonald & Jane's, 1976.

Bruyere, Rosallyn. *Wheels of Light, Chakras, Auras, and the Healing Energy of the Body*. New York: Fireside, 1989.

Byers, Dwight. *Better Health with Foot Reflexology*. Available through the International Institute of Reflexology, P.O. Box 12642, St. Petersburg, FL 33733-2642.

Chancellor, Phillip. *Handbook on the Bach Flower Remedies*. Keats, 1971.

Chocron, Daya Sarai. *Healing with Crystals and Gemstones*. York Beach, ME: Samuel Weiser Inc., 1983.

Clark, Linda. *The Ancient Art of Color Therapy*. Old Greenwich, CT: Devin-Adair Co., 1975.

Coulter, C. *Portraits of Homeopathic Medicine*. 2 vols. Berkeley: North Atlantic Books, 1986.

Cummings, Stephen, and Dana Ullman. *Everybody's Guide to Homeopathic Medicine*. Los Angeles: Jeremy P. Tarcher, 1991.

Gibson, D.M. *Studies of Homeopathic Remedies*. Beaconsfield, England: Beaconsfield Publishers, 1987.

Gimbel, Theo. *Healing with Color and Light*. London: Gaia Books, 1994.

Grof, Stanislav, M.D. *The Adventure of Self-Discovery: Dimensions of Consciousness and New Perspectives in Psychotherapy and Inner Exploration*. Albany, NY: State University of New York Press, 1984.

Grof, Stanislav, M.D., with Hal Z. Bennet. *The Holotropic Mind: The*

Three Levels of Human Consciousness and How They Shape Our Lives. San Francisco: HarperCollins, 1993.

Grossinger, Richard. *Homeopathy: An Introduction for Skeptics and Beginners.* Berkeley, CA: North Atlantic Books, 1993.

Hahnemann, Samuel. *The Organon of Medicine.* Translated by J. Kunli, A. Naude, and P. Pendleton. London: Gollancz, 1986.

Horan, Paula. *Empowerment Through Reiki: The Path to Personal and Global Transformation.* Wilmot, WI: Lotus Light Publications, 1992.

Krieger, Dolores. *Accepting Your Power to Heal: The Personal Practice of Therapeutic Touch.* Santa Fe, NM: Bear & Co., 1993.

———. *Therapeutic Touch: How to Use Your Hands to Help or to Heal.* Englewood Cliffs, NJ: Prentice-Hall, 1986.

———. *Living the Therapeutic Touch: Healing as a Lifestyle.* New York: Dodd, Mead, 1987.

Kunz, Kevin, and Barbara Kunz. *Complete Guide to Food Reflexology.* Rev. ed. Englewood Cliffs, NJ: Prentice-Hall, 1991.

———. *Hand and Foot Reflexology: A Self-Help Guide.* Englewood Cliffs, NJ: Prentice-Hall, 1984.

Lessell, Dr. Colin B. *The World Travellers' Manual of Homoeopathy.* Essex, England: CW Daniel Company Ltd., 1993.

Lockie, Andrew. *The Home Guide to Homeopathy.* New York: Simon & Schuster, 1989; 1993.

Macrae, Janet, Ph.D., R.N. *Therapeutic Touch: A Practical Guide.* New York: Knopf, 1987.

Mills, Simon, and Steven J. Finando. *Alternatives in Healing.* New York: New American Library, 1988.

Norman, Laura. *Feet First: A Guide to Foot Reflexology.* New York: Simon & Schuster, 1988.

Panos, Maesimund B. *Homeopathic Medicine at Home.* Los Angeles: Jeremy P. Tarcher, 1980.

Rose, Barry. *The Family Health Guide to Homeopathy.* Berkeley, CA: Celestial Arts, 1992.

Scheffer, Mechthild. *Bach Flower Therapy.* Inner Traditions, 1987.

SHEN Therapy Institute. *Information on Emotions, Your Body and SHEN Therapy.* Sausalito, CA: 1990.

Stein, Diane. *Healing with Gemstones and Crystals.* Freedom, CA: Crossing Press, 1996.

Stephenson, James H. *A Doctor's Guide to Helping Yourself with Homeopathic Remedies.* 1st British ed. Wellingborough, England: Thorsons Publishers, 1977.

Taylor, Kylea. *The Breathwork Experience: Exploration and Healing in*

Nonordinary States of Consciousness. Santa Cruz, CA: Hanford Mead, 1994.

Ullman, Dana. *Homeopathy: Medicine for the 21st Century.* Berkeley, CA: North Atlantic Books, 1988.

———. *Discovering Homeopathy.* Berkeley, CA: North Atlantic Books, 1991.

Vlamis, George. *Rescue Remedy.* London: HarperCollins, 1994.

Weiner, Michael. *The Complete Book of Homeopathy.* Garden City Park, NY: Avery Publishing Group, 1989.

Weinstein, Corey, and Nancy Bruning. *Healing Homeopathic Remedies.* New York: Dell Publishing, 1996.

Wills, Pauline. *The Reflexology Manual: An Easy-to-Use Illustrated Guide to the Healing Zones of the Hands and Feet.* Rochester, VT: Healing Arts Press, 1995.

Young, Phil. *The Art of Polarity Therapy: A Practitioner's Perspective.* Dorset, England: Prism Press, 1990.

HERBS AND HERBAL MEDICINE

BOOKS

Bergner, Paul. *The Healing Power of Ginseng and the Tonic Herbs.* Rocklin, CA: Prima Publishing, 1996.

Carroll, David. *The Complete Book of Natural Medicine.* New York: Summit Books, 1980.

Castleman, Michael. *The Healing Herbs.* Emmaus, PA: Rodale Press, 1991.

Elias, Jason, and Shelagh Masline. *Healing Herbal Remedies.* New York: Dell, 1995.

Hoffman, David. *The New Holistic Herbal.* Rockport, MA: Element Books, 1992.

Kloss, Jethro. *Back to Eden.* Rev. ed. Loma Linda, CA: Back to Eden Books Publishing Co., 1994.

Lucas, Richard M. *Miracle Medicine Herbs.* Englewood Cliffs, NJ: Prentice-Hall, 1990.

Mindell, Earl, R.Ph., Ph.D. *Earl Mindell's Herb Bible.* New York: Simon & Schuster, 1992.

Moore, Michael. *Medicinal Plants of the Desert and Canyon West.* Santa Fe, NM: Museum of New Mexico Press, 1989.

Murray, Michael T., N.D. *The Healing Power of Herbs.* Rocklin, CA: Prima Publishing, 1991.

————. *Natural Alternatives to Over-the-Counter and Prescription Drugs.* New York: William Morrow, 1994.

Ody, Penelope. *The Complete Medicinal Herbal.* New York: Dorling Kindersley, 1993.

Stein, Diane. *All Women Are Healers.* Freedom, CA: The Crossing Press, 1990.

Tierra, Lesley. *The Herbs of Life: Health and Healing Using Western and Chinese Techniques.* Freedom, CA: The Crossing Press, 1992.

————. *The Way of Herbs.* New York: Simon & Schuster, 1990.

Tietze, Harald. *Kombucha: The Miracle Fungus.* Wellow, UK: Gateway Books, 1995.

Trattler, Ross. *Better Health Through Natural Healing.* New York: McGraw-Hill, 1985.

Tyler, Varro E. *The Honest Herbal.* 3rd ed. Binghamton, NY: Haworth Press, 1993.

Weil, Andrew, M.D. *Natural Health, Natural Healing.* New York: Houghton Mifflin, 1990.

PERIODICALS

HerbalGram
American Botanical Council
P.O. Box 201660
Austin, TX 78720

Natural Health
Boston Common Press Limited Partnership
17 Station Street
Brookline, MA 02146
www.naturalhealth1.com

PRODUCTS

The Herb and Spice Collection
P.O. Box 118
Norway, IA 52318

Nature's Herbs
1010 46th Street
Emeryville, CA 94608

MASSAGE

BOOKS

Anhui Medical School, China. *Chinese Massage.* Point Roberts, WA: Hartley & Marks, 1987.

DePaoli, Carlo. *The Healing Touch of Massage*. New York: Sterling Publishing, 1995.

Harrold, Fiona. *The Complete Body Massage: A Hands-On Manual*. New York: Sterling Publishing, 1992.

Inkeles, Gordon. *The Art of Sensual Massage*. New York: Simon & Schuster, 1974.

Kaptchuk, Ted J. *The Web That Has No Weaver: Understanding Chinese Medicine*. New York: Congdon & Weed, 1993.

Lidell, Lucinda, et al. *The Book of Massage*. New York: Simon & Schuster, 1984.

Maxwell-Hudson, Clare. *The Complete Book of Massage*. New York: Random House, 1988.

Ravald, Bertild. *The Art of Swedish Massage*. New York: EP Dutton, 1984.

Sohn, Tina. *AMMA Therapy: An Integration of Oriental Medical Principles, Bodywork, Nutrition, & Exercise*. Rochester, VT: Inner Traditions, 1994.

Stillerman, Elaine. *Mothermassage: A Handbook for Relieving the Discomfort of Pregnancy*. New York: Delacorte, 1992.

Tappan, Frances M. *Healing Massage Techniques*. Stamford, CT: Appleton and Lange, 1988.

VIDEOS

Athletic Massage: Therapeutic Massage for Sports and Fitness
Rich Phaigh, CVT Productions
(800) 284-4403

Learn to Massage at Home
Well Aware Media
301 S. Bedford St.
Suite 212
Madison, WI 53703
(608) 255-5433

PERIODICAL

Massage magazine
P.O. Box 1500
Davis, CA 95617
(916) 757-6033

MIND THERAPIES

BOOKS

Alman, Brian M. *Self-Hypnosis: The Complete Manual*. New York: Brunner/Mazel, 1992.

Borysenko, Joan. *Minding the Body, Mending the Mind*. Toronto/New York: Bantam Books, 1988.

———. *The Power of the Mind to Heal*. Carson, CA: Hay House, 1994.

Brooks, Charles. *Sensory Awareness: The Rediscovery of Experiencing Through Workshops with Charlotte Selver*. Felix Morrow, 1986.

Copelan, Rachael. *How to Hypnotize Yourself and Others*. New York: Bell Publishing, 1984.

Cousins, Norman. *Anatomy of an Illness as Perceived by the Patient*. New York: Norton, 1979.

———. *Head First: The Biology of Hope and the Healing Power of the Human Spirit*. New York: Viking, 1990.

Dunham, Eileen, and Cindy Cooper. *Therapeutic Relaxation and Imagery Development Manual*. Cupertino, CA: Health Horizons, 1989.

Epstein, Gerald. *Healing Visualizations*. New York: Bantam, 1989.

Fanning, Patrick. *Visualization for Change*. Oakland, CA: New Harbinger, 1988.

Fezler, William. *Creative Imagery*. New York: Simon & Schuster, 1989.

Fisher, Stanley. *Discovering the Power of Self-Hypnosis*. New York: HarperCollins, 1991.

Goleman, Daniel, and Joel Gurin. *Mind Body Medicine: How to Use Your Mind for Better Health*. Yonkers, NY: Consumer Reports Books, 1993.

Green, Elmer. *Beyond Biofeedback*. New York: Delacorte, 1977.

Haley, Jay. *Uncommon Therapy*. New York: WW Norton, 1987. (hypnotherapy)

Hilgad, Ernest. *Hypnosis: In the Relief of Pain*. New York: Brunner/Mazel, 1994.

Kabat-Zinn, J. *Full Catastrophic Living: Using the Wisdom of Your Body and Mind to Face Stress, Pain, and Illness*. New York: Delacorte, 1990.

Klein, Allen. *The Healing Power of Humor*. Los Angeles: Jeremy P. Tarcher, 1989.

Lusk, Julie, ed. *30 Scripts for Relaxation, Imagery and Inner Healing*. 2 vols. Duluth, MN: Whole Person Associates, 1992.

McDonald, Kathleen. *How to Meditate*. Boston: Wisdom Publications, 1992.

Miller, Michael, M.D. *Therapeutic Hypnosis*. New York: Human Sciences Press, 1979.

Moen, Larry, ed. *Guided Imagery*. 2 vols. Naples: United States Publishing, 1992.

Moody, Raymond A. Jr., M.D. *Laugh After Laugh: The Healing Power of Humor*. Jacksonville, FL: Headwaters Press, 1978.

Naparstek, Belleruth. *Staying Well with Guided Imagery*. New York: Time / Warner, 1994.

Ornstein, Robert, and David Sobel. *The Healing Mind*. New York: Simon & Schuster, 1987.

Pelletier, Kenneth R. *Mind as Healer, Mind as Slayer*. Rev. ed. New York: Delacorte, 1992.

Rossman, Martin L., M.D. *Healing Yourself: A Step-by-Step Program for Better Health Through Imagery*. New York: Walker & Co., 1987.

Samuels, Michael, M.D. *Healing with the Mind's Eye: A Guide for Using Imagery and Visions for Personal Growth and Healing*. New York: Simon & Schuster, 1990.

Sedlacek, Kurt. *The Sedlacek Technique: Finding the Calm*. New York: McGraw-Hill, 1989. (biofeedback)

Siegel, Bernie S., M.D. *Peace, Love & Healing. Bodymind Communication and the Path to Self-Healing*. New York: Harper & Row, 1989.

————. *Love, Medicine and Miracles: Lessons Learned About Self-Healing From a Surgeon's Experience with Exceptional Patients*. Boston: GK Hall, 1988.

Wallace, Benjamin. *Applied Hypnosis*. Chicago: Nelson-Hall, 1979.

Weil, Andrew, M.D. *Spontaneous Healing*. Boston: Houghton Mifflin, 1994.

Yates, John. *The Complete Book of Self-Hypnosis*. Chicago: Nelson-Hall, 1984.

RESOURCES

Awareness and Relaxation Training
c/o Stress Reduction Program
Santa Cruz Medical Clinic
202 Soquel Avenue
Santa Cruz, CA 95062
(408) 458-5842

The Inner Art of Meditation by Jack Kornfield
The Present Moment: A Retreat on the Practice of Mindfulness, by Thich Nhat Hanh
Sounds True
(800) 333-9185
(each contains six audiocassettes)

Mind/Body Health Sciences Inc.
393 Dixon Road
Boulder, CO 80302
(*Circle of Healing* newsletter)

The Source Cassette Learning System
Emmet Miller, M.D.
945 Evelyn Street
Menlo Park, CA 94025
(415) 328-7171
(tapes for relaxation, pain relief; free catalog)

MISCELLANEOUS THERAPIES AND METHODS

BOOKS

Brint, Armand. "Iridology" in *The Holistic Health Handbook, 1978*. Edward Bauman, ed. Berkeley, CA: And/Or Press, 1978.

Garfield, Patricia. *The Healing Power of Dreams*. New York: Fireside/Simon & Schuster, 1992.

Harner, Michael. *The Way of the Shaman*. 3d ed. San Francisco: Harper San Francisco, 1990.

Kriege, Theodore. *Disease Signs in the Iris*. Romford, UK: LN Fowler, 1985.

LaBerge, Stephen. *Lucid Dreaming*. New York: Ballantine Books, 1985.

LaBerge, Stephen, and Howard Rheingold. *Exploring the World of Lucid Dreaming*. New York: Ballantine Books, 1990.

Lukeman, Alex. *What Your Dreams Can Teach You*. St. Paul, MN: Llewellyn Publications, 1990.

Mantell, Matthew. *Applied Kinesiology*. International College of Applied Kinesiology—USA. Shawnee Mission, KS: n.d.

Walker, Morton, DPM. *DMSO: Nature's Healer*. Stamford, CT: Avery Publishing, 1993.

AUDIOTAPES, LITERATURE

Bernard Jensen International
24360 Old Wagon Road
Escondido, CA 92027
(619) 749-2727
(Iridology)

MOVEMENT AND POSTURE THERAPIES

BOOKS

Alexander, F.M. *Constructive Conscious Control of the Individual*. Long Beach, CA: Centerline Press, 1985.

———. *Man's Supreme Inheritance*. Long Beach, CA: Centerline Press, 1989.

———. *The Use of the Self*. Long Beach, CA: Centerline Press, 1985.

———. *The Universal Constant in Living*. Long Beach, CA: Centerline Press, 1986.

Alexander, Gerda. *Eutony: The Holistic Discovery of the Total Person*. Felix Morrow, 1985. Available through Feldenkrais Resources, (800) 765-1907.

Anderson, Dale L., M.D. *90 Seconds to Muscle Pain Relief*. Minneapolis, MN: CompCare Publishers, 1992. (Fold and Hold)

Barlow, Wilfred, M.D. *The Alexander Technique: How to Use Your Body Without Stress*. Rochester, VT: Healing Arts Press, 1990.

Benjamin, Ben E. *Are You Tense? The Benjamin System of Muscular Therapy*. New York: Pantheon, 1978.

———. *Listen to Your Pain: Understanding, Identifying and Treating Pain and Injury*. New York: Viking Penguin, 1984.

Caplan, Deborah. *Back Trouble: A New Approach to Prevention and Recovery, Based on the Alexander Technique*. Gainesville, FL: Triad Publishing, 1987.

Clark, Barbara. *Jin Shin Acutouch: The Tai Chi of Healing Arts*. San Diego: Clark Publishing, 1987.

Cohen, Bonnie Bainbridge. *Sensing, Feeling, and Action: The Experiential Anatomy of Body-Mind Centering*. Contact Editions, 1993.

Dowd, Irene. *Taking Root to Fly: Articles on Functional Anatomy*. 3d ed. New York: Irene Dowd, 1995. (ideokinesis)

Feldenkrais, Moshe. *Awareness Through Movement: Easy-to-Do Health Exercises to Improve Your Posture, Vision, Imagination, & Personal Awareness*. San Francisco: Harper & Row, 1972.

———. *The Elusive Obvious or Basic Feldenkrais*. Cupertino, CA: Meta Publications, 1981.

Folan, Lilias. *Lilias, Yoga and Your Life*. New York: Macmillan, 1981.

Gray, John. *Your Guide to the Alexander Technique*. New York: St. Martin's Press, 1990.

Hartley, Linda. *Wisdom of the Body Moving: An Introduction to Body-Mind Centering*. Berkeley, CA: North Atlantic Books, 1995.

Hewitt, James. *The Complete Yoga Book*. New York: Schocken Books, 1978.

Juhan, Deane. *An Introduction to Trager Psychophysical Integration and Mentastics Movement Education*. Mill Valley, CA: The Trager Institute, 1989.

Knaster, Mirka. *Discovering the Body's Wisdom: A Comprehensive Guide to More than Fifty Mind-Body Practices*. New York: Bantam, 1996.

Knocking at the Gate of Life and Other Healing Exercises from China. Translated by Edward C. Chang. Emmaus, PA: Rodale Press, 1985.

Kundalini Research Institute. *Sadhana Guidelines for Kundalini Yoga Daily Practice*. Los Angeles: Arcline Publications, 1988.

Kuo, Simmone. *Long Life, Good Health through Tai-Chi Chuan*. Berkeley, CA: North Atlantic Books, 1991.

Lagerwerff, Ellen, and Karen Perlroth. *Mensendieck Your Posture and Your Pains*. New York: Aries, 1982.

Lee, Martin, and Emily Lee. *Ride the Tiger to the Mountain: Tai Chi for Health*. Reading, MA: Addison-Wesley, 1991.

Liebowitz, Judith, and Bill Connington. *The Alexander Technique: The World-Famous Method for Enhancing Posture, Stamina, Health, and Well-being, and for Relieving Pain and Tension*. New York: HarperCollins, 1990.

Liu, Hong, Dr. *Mastering Miracles: The Healing Art of Qi Gong as Taught by a Master*. New York: Time Warner, 1997.

Mensendieck, Bess. *The Mensendieck System of Functional Exercises*. Kristianstads Boktryckeri, 1989.

Monro, Robin, et al. *Yoga for Common Ailments*. New York: Simon & Schuster, 1990.

Rubenfeld, Ilana. "Gestalt Therapy and the BodyMind: An Overview of the Rubenfeld Synergy Method" in *Gestalt Therapy: Perspectives and Applications*. Edited by Edwin Nevis. New York: Gardner Press, 1992.

———. "Ushering in a Century of Integration" in *Somatics* Autumn/Winter 1990-91.

Saltonstall, Ellen. *Kinetic Awareness*. New York: Kinetic Awareness Center, 1988.

Sivananda Yoga Vedanta Center. *Learn Yoga in a Weekend*. New York: Knopf, 1993.

Sutton, Nigel. *Applied Tai Chi Chuan*. London: A&C Black, 1991.

Sweigard, Lulu E. *Human Movement Potential: Its Ideokinetic Facilitation*. New York: Dodd, Mead, 1975.

Trager, Milton, and C. Guadagno. *Trager Mentastics: Movement as a Way to Agelessness*. Barrytown, NY: Station Hill Press, 1987.

PERIODICALS

Yoga Journal
2054 University Avenue
Berkeley, CA 94704

VIDEOS AND RESOURCES

Feldenkrais Resources
830 Bancroft Way
Berkeley, CA 94710
(510) 540-7600

Mensendieck Academy and Enterprises
P.O. Box 9450
Stanford, CA 94309
(415) 851-8184
("Freedom from Back Pain: The Mensendieck System," video with booklet.)

The Healing Tao Center
P.O. Box 1194
Huntington, NY 11743
(516) 367-2701
(videos of *qigong* exercises)

Master Hong Inc.
P.O. Box 726
Duarte, CA 91009
(818) 359-7612 (fax)
(videos of *qigong*)

Physicalmind Institute
1807 Second Street, #281129
Santa Fe, NM 87505
(800) 505-1990
(videos on Pilates Method)

Samata Yoga and Health Institute
4150 Tivoli Avenue
Los Angeles, CA 90066
(310) 306-8845
(manuals, videos, and audiocassettes)

Healing Arts Publishing
321 Hampton Drive
Venice, CA 90291
("Tai Chi for Health" a two-hour video)

Yoga Journal
2054 University Avenue
Berkeley, CA 94704
("Yoga for Beginners")

The School for Body-Mind Centering
189 Pondview Drive
Amherst, MA 01002
(413) 256-8615
(videos and books)

NATUROPATHY

BOOKS

MacEoin. *Healthy by Nature*. London: HarperCollins, 1994.

Turner, Roger Newman. *Naturopathic Medicine*. London: Thorsons, HarperCollins, 1990.

NUTRITIONAL AND SUPPLEMENTAL THERAPIES

BOOKS

Balch, James F., and Phyllis Balch. *Prescription for Nutritional Healing*. Garden City Park, NY: Avery Publishing Group, 1993.

Ballentine, Rudolph. *Transition to Vegetarianism: An Evolutionary Step*. Honesdale, PA: Himalayan Publishers, 1987.

Carper, Jean. *Food—Your Miracle Medicine*. New York: HarperCollins, 1993.

Colbin, Annemarie. *Food and Healing*. New York: Ballantine, 1986.

Foster, Steven. *Echinacea: Nature's Immune Enhancer*. Rochester, VT: Healing Arts Press, 1991.

Fulder, Stephen, and John Blackwood. *Garlic: Nature's Original Remedy*. Rochester, VT: Healing Arts Press, 1991.

Haas, Elson M., M.D. *Staying Healthy with Nutrition*. Berkeley, CA: Celestial Arts, 1992.

Haas, Robert. *Eat Smart, Think Smart*. New York: HarperCollins, 1994.

Haught, S.J. *The American Experience of Dr. Max Gerson*. Bonita, CA: The Gerson Institute, 1991.

Hendler, Sheldon Saul, M.D. *The Complete Guide to Anti-Aging Nutrients*. New York: Simon & Schuster, 1985.

Hobbs, Christopher. *Medicinal Mushrooms*. Capitola, CA: Botanica Press, 1986.

Hoffer, Abram, Ph.D., and Morton Walker, D.P.M. *Smart Nutrients*. Garden City Park, NY: Avery Publishing, 1994.

Kaiser, Jon D., M.D. *Immune Power*. New York: St. Martin's Press, 1993.

Klaper, Michael, M.D. *Vegan Nutrition Pure and Simple*. Maui, HI: Gentle World, 1987.

Lappe, Frances M. *Diet for a Small Planet*. Rev. ed. New York: Ballantine Books, 1975.

McDougall, John M., M.D. *McDougall's Medicine*. Piscataway, NJ: New Century, 1985.

Null, Gary, Ph.D., and Marvin Feldman, M.D. *Reverse the Aging Process Naturally*. New York: Villard Books, 1993.

Ohsawa, George. *The Art of Peace*. Oroville, CA: George Ohsawa Macrobiotic Foundation, 1990.

Passwater, Richard, Ph.D. *The Antioxidants*. New Canaan, CT: Keats Publishing, 1985.

Pitchford, Paul. *Healing with Whole Foods: Oriental Traditions and Modern Nutrition*. Berkeley, CA: North Atlantic Books, 1993.

Reuben, Carolyn. *Antioxidants: Your Complete Guide*. Rocklin, CA: Prima Publishing, 1995.

Robbins, John. *Diet for a New America: How Your Food Choices Affect Your Health, Happiness, and the Future of Life on Earth*. Walpole, NH: Stillpoint Publishing, 1987.

———. *May All Be Fed*. New York: Morrow, 1992; Avon, 1993.

Theodosakis, Jason M.D., M.S., M.P.H., Brenda Adderly, M.H.A. & Barry Fox, Ph.D. *The Arthritis Cure*. New York: St. Martin's Press, 1997.

Wasserman, Debbie. *Simply Vegan: Quick Vegetarian Meals*. Baltimore: Vegetarian Resource Group, 1991.

Werbach, Melvyn. *Healing Through Nutrition*. New York: HarperCollins, 1993.

White, J.R., and R.K. Campbell. "Magnesium and diabetes: A review" in *Ann Pharmacother* 27: 775-80, 1993.

PERIODICALS/RESOURCES

Natural Hygiene, Inc.
P.O. Box 2132
Huntington, CT 06484
(203) 929-1557
(publishes *The Journal of Natural Hygiene*)

North American Vegetarian Society
P.O. Box 72
Dodgerville, NY 13329
(518) 568-7970
(publishes *The Vegetarian Voice* magazine)

The McDougall Program
P.O. Box 14039
Santa Rosa, CA 95402
(707) 576-1654

The Nutrition Action Health Letter
Center for Science in the Public Interest
1875 Connecticut Avenue NW, Suite 300
Washington, DC 20009-5728
(202) 332-9111
(monthly newsletter for the general public)

Physicians Committee for Responsible Medicine
P.O. Box 6322
Washington, DC 20015
(202) 686-2210
(publishes *Good Medicine* magazine)

Vegetarian Times
P.O. Box 570
Oak Park, IL 60303
(708) 848-8100
(monthly publication)

PHYSICAL THERAPIES

Northrup, G.D. *Osteopathic Medicine: An American Reformation, 2nd edition.* Chicago: American Osteopathic Association, 1979.

Upledger, John E., D.O., O.M.M. *CranioSacral Therapy, Somato-Emotional Release, Your Inner Physician and You.* Berkeley, CA: North Atlantic Books; and Palm Beach Gardens, FL: The Upledger Institute, 1991.

PSYCHOLOGICAL THERAPIES

Collingwood, C., and J. Collingwood. *Personal Strategies for Life: A Practitioners' Manual for Students of NLP.* Sydney, Australia: Inspiritive Party Ltd., 1995.

Dilts, R., et al. *Neuro-Linguistic Programming: The Study of the Structure of Subjective Experience.* Vol. 1. Cupertino, CA: Meta Publications, 1980.

Janov, Arthur. *The New Primal Scream: Primal Therapy Twenty Years On.* Wilmington, DE: Enterprise Publishing, 1991.

Netherton, Morris, and Nancy Shiffrin. *Past Lives Therapy*. New York: William Morrow, 1978.

Orr, Leonard, and Sandra Ray. *Rebirthing in the New Age*. Berkeley, CA: Celestial Arts, 1983.

Ray, Sandra. *Celebration of Breath: Rebirthing, Book I*. Berkeley, CA: Celestial Arts, 1983.

SENSORY THERAPIES

BOOKS

Goodrich, Janet, Ph.D. *Natural Vision Improvement*. Berkeley, CA: Celestial Arts, 1985.

Lavabre, Marcel. *The Aromatherapy Workbook*. Rochester, VT: Healing Arts Press, 1990.

Leviton, Richard. *Seven Steps to Better Vision*. Brookline, MA: East West/Natural Health Books, 1992.

Merritt, Stephanie. *Mind, Music, and Imagery*. New York: Plume Press, 1990.

Rose, Jeanne. *The Aromatherapy Book*. Berkeley, CA: North Atlantic Books, 1992.

Taber, Jerriann. *Eye-Robics*. El Cajon, CA: Vision Training Institute, n.d.

Tomatis, Alfred. *The Conscious Ear*. Staton Hill Books, 1991.

Worwood, Valerie Ann. *The Complete Book of Essential Oils and Aromatherapy*. San Rafael, CA: New World Library, 1991.

PRODUCTS

Aroma-Vera, Inc.
5901 Rodeo Road
Los Angeles, CA 90016-43112
(800) 669-9514

Original Swiss Aromatics
P.O. Box 6842
San Rafael, CA 94903
(415) 459-3998

Santa Fe Fragrance
P.O. Box 282
Santa Fe, NM 87504

Windrose Aromatics
12629 N. Tatum Blvd., Suite 611
Phoenix, AZ 85032

Treat depression naturally with "Nature's Prozac"—learn the...

SECRETS
of
St. JOHN'S WORT

LARRY KATZENSTEIN

St. John's wort is the miracle herb that's making headlines with its amazing healing properties. If you suffer from depression, anxiety, insomnia or SAD, and don't want the expense or unpleasant side-effects of prescription drugs, it may be just what you're looking for. Find out in this exhaustive, well-researched, and easy-to-use volume.

SECRETS OF ST. JOHN'S WORT
Larry Katzenstein
0-312-96574-5___$5.99 U.S.___$7.99 Can.

Publishers Book and Audio Mailing Service
P.O. Box 070059, Staten Island, NY 10307
Please send me the book(s) I have checked above. I am enclosing $_____ (please add $1.50 for the first book, and $.50 for each additional book to cover postage and handling. Send check or money order only—no CODs) or charge my VISA, MASTERCARD, DISCOVER or AMERICAN EXPRESS card.

Card Number_____

Expiration date_____Signature_____
Name_____
Address_____
City_____State/Zip_____
Please allow six weeks for delivery. Prices subject to change without notice. Payment in U.S. funds only. New York residents add applicable sales tax.   STJOHN 3/98